Sweet Deceptions

Sweet Deceptions

CREATE DECADENT DESSERTS
WITHOUT ALL THAT FAT (OR GUILT)!

Patty Neeley

———

PRIMA PUBLISHING

PRIMA PUBLISHING and colophon are trademarks of Prima Communications, Inc.

Library of Congress Cataloging-in-Publication Data

Neeley, Patty Ann.
    Sweet Deceptions : create decadent desserts without all that fat (or guilt)! / by Patty Ann Neeley.
        p.   cm.
    Includes index.
    ISBN 0-7615-0287-4
    1. Desserts.   2. Low-fat diet—Recipes.   I. Title.
TX733.N38   1996
641.8'6—dc20   95-42385
                                                                                                        CIP

96 97 98 99 00 AA 10 9 8 7 6 5 4 3 2 1
Printed in the United States of America

How to Order:

Single copies may be ordered from Prima Publishing, P.O. Box 1260BK, Rocklin, CA 95677; telephone (916) 632-4400. Quantity discounts are also available. On your letterhead, include information concerning the intended use of the books and the number of books you wish to purchase.

This book is dedicated to my husband, Randy Stahlberger.
I am very fortunate to have such a positive driving force behind me.
Only great things can happen when we work together as a team,
as I have discovered every day since you came into my life.
I love you, Randy.

Life is Uncertain,
Eat Dessert First!

Contents

Contents

Special Thanks

Several great people are responsible for the successful completion of *Sweet Deceptions*. I would like to take this
opportunity to thank my wonderfully supportive friends for
their constant belief in my ability to pull this project off, and
especially for helping me chip away at what seemed like an endless supply of cookies, muffins, and desserts from all of the
recipe testing.

This book would not have materialized without the un-
wavering support of Prima Publishing. What a fantastic team. I
want to thank each and every person there for their part in
bringing this manuscript to book form—especially the ones who
had to edit my completed manuscript!

To Georgia Hughes: Thank you for seeing my vision for
this book. A huge thanks for your time and patience (especially
when it came to that return button!)—may we do many more
books together in the future!

To the book cover dream team: photographer Kent Lacin,
props extraordinaire Greta Lacin, cover design specialist Lindy
Dunlavey, and food stylist Patty Mastracco. Thank you for your
incredible creativity and devotion to your work!

To my grandmother, Dorothea Skailand: Thanks, Gramma,
for setting me on my culinary path all those years ago, and for
teaching me that honesty and hard work truly do get rewarded.
I think those eggshells in the cake were a sign!

To Joyce Marie Greer: Thank you from the bottom of my heart for your unconditional love and support. A big thanks to Bill and Betty Stahlberger for all of your encouragement and support. To my very close friends Ann Lange and crazy Dave: May the sun shine on your lives and bring you the warmth you have brought to me. I love you both very much and will never be able to fully express my gratitude for the love and support you gave me through a rough time in my life.

And finally, I would like to say a very special thank you to Ben and Nancy Dominitz, not only for your help and support for my book endeavor, but for your belief in me and my abilities as a chef. Our experiences together over the last two years have not only inspired great food, but have also brought out abilities that I never really believed I had, and for that I am forever grateful.

Introduction

My motivation for writing this book springs from my sweet tooth and the ongoing need to satisfy it!

Throughout my years in the restaurant business, I have both created and indulged in some of the most sinful, gooey, and wickedly chocolate desserts imaginable, and I shamelessly devoured each and every one with reckless abandon and total disregard for the consequences, measured, of course, in pounds and inches. I enjoyed every last, luscious bite right down to licking the plate clean when any watchful eyes were looking the other way.

If this secret life sounds all too familiar to you, join me now in my confession: "I am a devout dessert lover—always have been, always will be!" Unfortunately, desserts worth eating are almost always very fattening and high in calories. So here we are, caught smack dab in the middle of this health-conscious age, and those decadent creations that we love so much are all but forbidden except for the occasional splurge or special event.

Even so, I continue to crave fabulous sweets on a regular basis, and find myself unfulfilled by the ultra-lowfat and fat-free dessert options that are available these days. From store-bought items to lowfat recipes that claim to have great flavor and texture, I can find no sincere gratification. My longing for the real thing cannot be satisfied by desserts made of tofu and wheat germ. I want something I can really sink my sweet tooth into. Give me decadence or give me death! . . . or you can just give me Death by Chocolate if you like.

With all that in mind, I quickly became inspired to make a difference and completely dispel the myth that lowfat means no flavor and consequently no fun. I was on a quest to get as close to the real thing as possible and still maintain an acceptable level of calories and fat grams. Fueled by dreams of chocolate tortes and creamy custards and the nightmares of never getting enough of them, I have created a worthy selection of lower fat, lower calorie desserts, from simple tea-time cookies and bars and moist fudgy-textured brownies to some of the most decadent to-die-fors like Tiramisù and Chocolate Raspberry Sanctuary. What's that? You can't believe what you're reading? Welcome to my sweet, deceptive world. You may still have a hard time believing, especially after you've sunk your sweet tooth into a Turtle Brownie that has been splashed with gooey caramel and toasted pecans!

Mind you, this book is not for the absolute health fanatic. Personally I have never found anything even remotely satisfying in a completely fat-free, ultra-low-calorie dessert. When it comes to desserts, I believe that just cutting back on the calories and fat grams is quite an achievement on its own, and will make a significant and positive impact on one's diet. This book is my answer to those unquenchable cravings for such things as New York-style cheesecake and creamy crème brûlée!

The recipes in this book are my best lowfat interpretations of classic desserts and treats, as well as some new creations. I find it extremely important to feel as though I am eating the real thing, and not some tasteless, lifeless, lowfat *wannabe*. I worked carefully with the chemistry of the ingredients to create that "mouth feel" that we depend on so much when we eat desserts, so don't be surprised at all when you find recipes for gooey caramel sauce, satiny crème anglaise (vanilla custard sauce), and rich dark-chocolate ganache. And by all means, feel free to use the Finishing Touches recipes to garnish desserts throughout the book for that extra-decadent touch, without the extra-decadent calories and fat grams.

I have done my best to keep the ingredients simple and familiar, with the exception of a few specialty items that can be found at gourmet food stores or delicatessens. As for the recipes themselves, you'll find the majority of them reasonably easy to follow and not too time-consuming. Who has the patience to wait through two hours of prep time and another hour of baking plus cooling time on top of that before they can sit down, relax, and have their just desserts? I have included, however, a few more involved and time-consuming recipes for those dinner parties or special occasions. Besides, Death by Chocolate never came from a half hour of work!

Right about now I'll bet you can hardly wait to flip these pages to try the first recipe. Better yet, you can hardly wait to taste these goodies! With great self-restraint I am resisting the temptation to tell you which treats will thrill you the most, and make the hair on your neck stand on end, but I do offer a hint to all the Tiramisù fanatics out there—satisfaction lurks only a few chapters away!

So come out of that closet and hand over those full-fat candy bars . . . and those cupcakes too! *Sweet Deceptions* is going to change the way you feel about the best part of life, DESSERT!

Sweet Deceptions

Chapter One

General Baking Tips and Helpful Hints

I think every cookbook ought to have a section of general baking tips. Naturally, many things about cooking and baking go without saying, but every cookbook author is different, therefore every recipe and method will be somewhat different, too. That's why I've opted to pass along some information that I feel would be greatly to your advantage when using this particular book. I know that baking in general can be quite an adventure on its own without throwing in this lower-fat ratio which can really affect the outcome of certain recipes. This chapter includes *general* helpful hints and information, and as you read through the book you will find a list of helpful hints at the beginning of each chapter that pertain to those particular recipes. Between these two resources, you're sure to find the answer you're looking for. And so without further ado . . .

Combining Dry Ingredients

I have found a wire whisk very useful for combining dry ingredients after measuring them into a bowl. I don't often require you to sift them, and the wire whisk helps to break up any lumps in the flour, sugar, cornstarch, etc.

1

Mixers and Mixing Methods

For these recipes, I haven't made any great demands when it comes to the type of electric mixer to use. Although I have had a heavy-duty KitchenAid stand mixer at my constant disposal since my graduation from culinary school ten years ago, you don't need to go out and buy one in order to execute the techniques in this book. However, if you are the proud owner of one of these great machines, by all means feel free to use it!

When I created the recipes for this book, I wanted to maintain a sense of simplicity. I mentally put myself in the average household kitchen just long enough to snoop around and take note of the type of equipment available. At the top of my list was the trusty hand-held mixer, which just about everybody has these days. So I went out and bought a good quality hand-held mixer and decided that I was going to make every recipe using it. The only exception is the stiffer cookie doughs. You may have to use a little elbow grease to mix them completely, unless your hand mixer is more up-to-date with an attachable dough hook or a paddle made specifically for heavy cookie doughs. I'm passing this information on to you in case you were ready to go out and spend $250 on a heavy-duty stand mixer. You will find more information on mixers in the equipment section of the next chapter.

Egg White and Meringue Tips

If you have ever beaten egg whites or made meringue, then you know firsthand what a chore it can be! Sometimes my meringue couldn't come out more beautifully. Other times I've spent long afternoons scrubbing the sticky mess off the wall (I think we all know how and why it got there). I wish it wasn't such a temperamental thing to make, but the rewards are so great when all goes well, that it's worth the effort.

The first thing to keep in mind is that if it's a sticky, muggy, humid day, you may as well forget it! Put those eggs back in the fridge, pour yourself a tall, cool one, and take the day off! Many

recipes fall victim to the weather and it's better just to make it another day rather than put yourself through the nightmare of trying
to overcome nature.

On normal baking days, the most important rule to remember
is that your egg whites have to be at room temperature if you ex-
pect to get decent volume out of them. You have probably read this
rule in every baking book imaginable; it is very important. It can
mean the difference of up to a quarter of the volume in your
meringue. Because baking a cake can be a very spontaneous act, we
sometimes need to take shortcuts. I have the best solution around.
Crack your egg whites into a mixing bowl and set that over
another bowl filled with hot, not boiling, water. With a clean and
grease-free utensil, stir the whites around a bit until they feel
slightly warm to the touch, just above room temperature. This
warmth allows the whites to achieve maximum volume when you
beat them.

On the subject of clean and grease-free, not only should your
egg whites be free of any impurities like bits of yolk, but the bowl
you beat them in and the beaters too should be squeaky clean. Any
trespassers can keep the whites from whipping up.

When beating the egg whites, always make sure that they have
reached soft peaks before starting to add the sugar. I have found
that bringing them up to soft peaks on a slower speed, such as
medium, helps preserve and strengthen the air pockets in the
meringue before you add the sugar. Once the whites have reached
the soft-peak stage you can increase the mixer speed to high and
begin to sprinkle in the sugar. Add about a tablespoon at a time
while continuing to beat and move the beaters around the bowl to
distribute the sugar. Keep sprinkling in the sugar continuously as
each tablespoon is absorbed into the meringue. When all the sugar
has been added the mixture should be stiff and glossy. Do not continue to beat it once it has reached this stage.

Now the mixture is ready to be baked as a crisp meringue or
folded into other ingredients. When folding meringue into another
batter, always use a delicate hand so as not to deflate the batter. For
the greatest success, fold with a rubber spatula, carefully lifting the

mixture up from the bottom of the bowl with a rolling movement. Make sure that there are no streaks of white and that the batter is uniform. Never tap the pan on the counter to level the batter; just carefully smooth the top with the spatula before putting the pan in the oven.

About Those Ovens!

If every oven in the world were the same make and model and in perfect calibration all the time, then I obviously would not need to slip this section into my book. In reality we're far from living in a perfect world. Unfortunately our ovens seem to have minds of their own, especially when we are trying to bake something in them! However, if you are the owner of one of those really nice, perfectly calibrated, state-of-the-art ovens that are precise to the very degree, I envy you! You probably won't have too much trouble in this department. As for the rest of us, believe it or not there is hope. I'll have you know this book was not put together with the help of a fancy test kitchen with all the latest gadgets. In fact, it was just the opposite. I had the joy of working with my very own, very average, temperamental-at-times oven, which more than qualifies me to understand any problems that such ovens can cause.

Right off the bat, remember that suggested oven times and temperatures are just that—suggestions! Usually I have found them to be fairly accurate, within five minutes or less of the actual baking time it took. Of course those were the times when my own oven was having a reasonably accurate day itself. Nevertheless, I have developed the habit of peeking in on things when they are within ten minutes of completion according to the recipe. This rule does change a bit for those items that have a much shorter baking time, like fifteen to twenty minutes. I wait until the last five minutes of baking time to check on these goodies.

As for baking temperatures, these depend greatly on the accuracy of your oven. If your oven has the unfortunate and often annoying problem that mine does of baking consistently too high or too low by let's say 25 degrees Fahrenheit, you can easily adjust it accordingly. An oven thermometer is well worth the investment for checking the actual temperature, which will make a tremendous difference in the outcome of the recipes.

Always trust your best judgment. After all, you're the one in control, not the oven! Paying close attention to how things should look and feel to the touch when they are done will be your best guard against mistakes.

What the Heck Is a Cake Tester?

Way back when, we used to say, "Stick a toothpick in the center to test for doneness." Well, I guess we've come a long way because now we have cake testers. I find these gizmos to be nothing more than glorified, expensive toothpicks! I bought one once to see if it was any better than the long bamboo skewers that I keep in the utensil drawer for testing my cakes. The official tester I got was a long piece of wire with a loop on the end to hold when sticking it into the cake. I found it a bit on the flimsy side, but some people wouldn't dream of using anything else. So my point is that when I use the term "cake tester," I mean anything suitable for sticking into a cake to check it, from toothpicks and bamboo skewers to "official" cake testers. As for using them properly, in my recipe instructions I have asked you to bake for the allotted time or until a cake tester inserted into the center comes out clean. This direction simply means to insert the tester into the center of the cake when it is close to being done or at the end of the allotted time. Withdraw it to see whether it comes out with batter on it, a clean tester indicates it's done.

The Hot-Knife Method for Cutting Desserts

Have you ever baked a really nice cake or a fudgy batch of brownies only to tear it up when you tried to cut it? This doesn't happen with every cake or bar-type dessert, but there are the exceptions, and for those times when you definitely want to get a nice clean cut without turning the whole dessert inside out with each slice of the

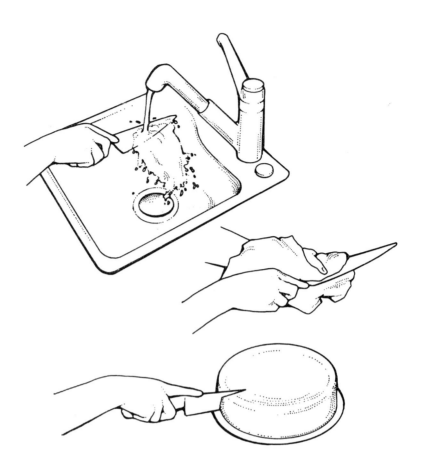

knife, I'd like to suggest the very successful hot-knife method. Nothing works better when you're dealing with something very moist like cheesecake or fudgy and gooey brownies. All you do is run a sharp knife under very hot water to heat the blade and immediately wipe it dry before cutting your dessert. You should repeat the process every time you make a new cut. I have found it especially helpful to leave the knife a little damp when cutting brownies, as doing so helps to keep crumbs from sticking to the knife.

I hope my list of helpful hints will answer any questions that may arise as you bake from this book. Remember, pay attention to

Sweet Deceptions

the little things, and use your best judgment and your own creativity to have a fantastic baking experience. I want to remind everyone, including myself, about three simple things before we embark on our great baking journey:

Always anticipate the room temperature rule indicated for certain recipes; it is easy to overlook. You can save precious time instead of waiting for an ingredient to come to room temperature.

Read all of the instructions before beginning anything. No one likes nasty surprises, especially not me, and reading all the way to the end of the recipe is the best way to avoid them.

And last but not least . . . HAVE FUN!

Chapter Two

Equipment and Special Ingredients

Equipment

Equipment is very important when it comes to baking and cooking, but I don't require the most exotic things on the market in order to execute my recipes. If you are an experienced cook or baker and have any of those fancy cake or tart pans and fluted pudding molds, then I would certainly encourage you to use them. But if you don't, the fanciest things you may need to purchase will be some ceramic or glass ramekins, and a tart pan with a removable bottom, which are easy to get ahold of these days. Please read the following list of equipment I have used to prepare these recipes. I include only those things which may require some explanation or offer helpful hints from my experience.

Electric Mixer

I have mentioned that I made all the recipes for this book using a simple handheld mixer. If you have a stand mixer, great; otherwise a hand mixer will work just fine. There are many brands to choose from these days, if you happen to be going out to buy one. I have a nice little mixer called Chef Mate, made by West Bend. I chose it not only because it has a wide range of speed settings, but because it has several other attachments such as flat beaters and dough hooks. So far it has stood up to every kind of dough and batter that I have mixed with it. There are also many other fine hand mixers made by such companies as Black & Decker and KitchenAid.

Food Processor

If you are serious at all about cooking or baking, then you know that it is next to impossible to get by without one of these. You will need a food processor to do many of the recipes in this book, but it does not have to be top of the line or even full-size. I have very limited cooking space, so I bought a smaller-size food processor. It is called the Little Pro Plus, made by Cuisinart. With a capacity of about four cups, it has all the power and performance of the big guys, and it takes up half the space. Any brand will do for the recipes in this book, but if you have to go buy one I would strongly suggest investing in one that will meet all of your cooking and baking demands.

Baking Pans

This is no ordinary baking book; therefore any old pan just won't do. I learned this lesson the hard way when I tried baking some of the cakes in nonstick bakeware and found they were very susceptible to burning. I have had the best luck with glass/Pyrex and heavier aluminum bakeware. All the round cakes were baked in aluminum cake pans made by companies like Wilton and Magic Line.

Cake and Loaf Pans

The cake pan sizes you will need are 8, 9, and 10 inches across and 2 inches deep. I have noticed that cake pans vary in depth and this can be crucial to the success of a recipe, so please check the depth before you begin. All of the loaf cakes were baked in aluminum or glass pans, size 8 × 3 3/4 inches. The other pans needed are an 8-inch square pan and a 9 × 13-inch rectangular pan, either glass or aluminum.

Bundt Pans

Be sure to use a standard size, 10 inches across, preferably aluminum. Double-check the size, because there are a couple of smaller sizes available.

Sweet Deceptions

Springform Pans

There are five cheesecakes in this book, and unless you have a springform pan, you won't be sinking your sweet tooth into any of them! If you are unfamiliar with this type of pan, it is round, ranging in size from 6 inches across to as wide as 14 inches. The sizes you will be using for this book are 8, 9, and 10 inches across by 3 inches deep. The pan is composed of two parts, the top piece is an adjustable ring with a spring-loaded latch, and the bottom fits snugly into the groove of the ring. The latch snaps closed, holding the bottom in place. After a cheesecake has been baked and cooled and is ready to serve, you simply unlatch the side and remove the ring, leaving the cheesecake on the bottom of the pan. These pans are also used for other types of cakes. We've come a long way when it comes to springform pans. I remember times when I had to hunt all over town to pick up a springform pan because the one I had was missing the top or bottom or just plain missing! Now you can find them in a number of different stores, and there are several types to choose from. They range in price from the really cheap and flimsy to the heavy-duty SilverStone-lined, "Why would I pay that much money for a springform!" type. I have always gotten the best performance out of the middle-of-the-road, somewhat heavy, and well made aluminum springform pan.

Tart Pans

The collection of desserts in this book would have been incomplete without a few tarts. For these you will need a 9-inch fluted tart pan with removable bottom, made of aluminum or stainless steel. You can find one at a specialty cooking and baking shop. What differentiates this type of pan from the springform pan is that it is very shallow, about an inch deep, and there is no latch. Instead the bottom simply rests on the wide inner lip of the side ring. To unmold the tart, you just push the bottom plate up from underneath and it comes right out.

Cookie Sheets

I want to mention again that nonstick bakeware does not work well for the recipes in this book. You'll get much better results from a heavy aluminum sheet pan. If you have access to a restaurant supply store, you would do well to purchase an aluminum half sheet pan, which is a bit larger than a regular cookie sheet. It will last just about forever and tends to warp less than thinner sheet pans do.

Custard Cups and Pudding Molds

Several types of molds can be used for desserts, but the most practical are 5-ounce ceramic or glass ramekins. These look exactly like large soufflé dishes and can be used for all of the custards and puddings in this book. If you like to entertain and would like to serve your lowfat crème brûlée in something other than a white ramekin, shop around a bit. I have seen ramekins in different colors, some with beautiful flowers and other designs painted on them. I even found some great earthenware ones in a little antique store once, and I am always checking thrift shops and flea markets—in fact, that's how I acquired a lot of my equipment!

Saucepans

Always use heavy-bottomed pans for good, even heat conductivity; you will be less likely to scorch a mixture. Stainless steel is one of the best ways to go, other than professional-style cookware made of anodized steel. Enamel-coated cast-iron pans are also a good choice.

Muffin Pans

I like to use aluminum pans. You'll probably want one full pan (12) and one half pan (6), since most of these recipes make 12–16 muffins.

Mixing Bowls

The type of bowl you use to mix ingredients in may not seem important, yet the bowl can be critical to the success of certain recipes. Stainless steel, copper, or a sturdy, Pyrex-type glass are the best choices. Not only are they squeaky clean after a good washing (essential for making meringue), they are made especially for mixing with an electric mixer or a wire whisk. Ceramic bowls, as pretty as they can be to look at, can be ruined on the inside by electric mixers or whisks. I have even seen some chip from the spinning beaters. It's better to use the stainless steel bowls, which are made to take the abuse!

Utensils

Candy Thermometer

Made of glass or metal, these are manufactured specifically for making candy and have a range of 400° with markers for jelly, soft ball, hard ball, and hard crack.

Wire Whisk

I consider a whisk to be one of the most indispensable tools in my kitchen. I have several, in a range of sizes. Now you don't have to have a whisk collection, but you really should have at least one good wire whisk. Avoid cheap ones with only four flimsy wires. At a quality kitchenware shop purchase a stainless steel, elongated balloon whisk that measures about 8 inches from the base of the wires to the tip. It should have at least eight wires. That is the size of the one that I used while creating the recipes in this book and it worked perfectly for every little task. The reason I use the elongated whisk is for the convenience of being able to switch to a smaller bowl without having to change whisk sizes. You'll find that the 8-inch whisk works quite well in any kind of bowl.

Fine-mesh Sieve

If you plan to make any of the pureed fruit sauces in Finishing Touches, then you will want to have one of these tools on hand, especially if you hate berry seeds as much as I do. The wire mesh is much finer than the standard wire strainer so it can keep those tiny little seeds out of your sauce while allowing all the liquid and vital pulp to pass through. These sieves are also fantastic for dusting cakes and desserts with cocoa or powdered sugar since the finer mesh controls the amount of sugar or cocoa that goes through.

Metal Icing Spatulas

You'll find these tools quite invaluable once you realize they're good for more than just icing cakes. I use mine for everything from the obvious to lifting cookies off sheet pans, transferring cakes from one place to another, smoothing batters, and about a thousand other tasks. There are two kinds of spatulas: flat and angled. Both types will be quite useful to you for making these recipes. They come in an abundance of sizes; the ones I use the most are a 6-inch flat and an 8-inch angled spatula.

Parchment Paper

I use this paper religiously whenever I am working in a restaurant, but at home it's much easier to reach for the roll of aluminum foil. Parchment paper is made specifically to withstand the heat of the oven, so you can line all of your cake pans and cookie sheets with it instead of foil. I haven't, however, found a good source of parchment for home baking. When I can find it, it comes in an obnoxious roll that you have to cut and somehow coax to flatten. If you have access to a box of parchment sheets, then I strongly encourage you to use parchment instead of foil, especially for baking meringues, but I do not require it for these recipes.

Cardboard Cake Circles

These simple items really come in handy for a number of purposes, first and foremost for removing a dessert from the pan it was baked in, so you can wash the pan and not cut on it. If you want to put your cake or tart on a serving plate, these cardboard disks can help you transfer it without batting an eyelash. If you need to refrigerate or even freeze cake layers, these disks are perfect to put them on before wrapping in plastic. This procedure ensures that your layers are supported and will not warp or crack. Cake circles come in a wide range of sizes, but for the desserts in this book I used a 10-inch round. You can find them anywhere that sells cake-decorating supplies, as well as some specialty cookware and bakeware shops.

Special Ingredients

These recipes are full of many common ingredients, but some others may need a bit of explanation, either about where to find them, or if there are acceptable substitutions for them. I have gone through and picked out the ingredients that I feel most require elaboration.

Dairy

Butter: I use light butter, a lighter version of the real thing, made with ingredients like buttermilk and gelatin in order to reduce the fat grams and calories. Most brands indicate that they are not recommended for baking or frying, but I found light butter to be quite satisfactory for my recipes. The brands I used are Challenge and Land O' Lakes, each having approximately 50 calories and 6 grams of fat per tablespoon.

Cottage cheese: I like to use lowfat small-curd cottage cheese that has 2 percent milk fat. Each 1-ounce serving contains approximately 26 calories and 1/2 gram of fat.

Liquid nondairy creamer: This ingredient was designed to take the place of milk and light cream. I chose to use it in certain recipes instead of light cream because it has no saturated fat and no cholesterol. Look for it unsweetened and unflavored. Each tablespoon should have approximately 20 calories and 1.5 grams of fat.

Mascarpone cheese: This rich Italian cream cheese gives Tiramisù its unmistakable texture and taste. You can find it in gourmet food shops and delicatessens. I have also seen it in the cheese section of some grocery stores. Always taste it first. It should not be sour and should have a creamy texture. Any sign of graininess or separation is an indication of an inferior product that may also be old. Always check the expiration date on the bottom of the container.

Neufchâtel cheese: This is very similar to cream cheese, and the light version is excellent for making lower fat cheesecakes and other desserts. It is not fat-free, but is reduced in fat by a third, containing 70 calories and 6 grams of fat per ounce. There are many brands of reduced-fat cream cheese on the market, but I prefer Philadelphia-brand cream cheese for its quality and creaminess. You can use any brand, as long as the calories and fat grams are close to what I've indicated above.

Nondairy whipped topping: This product is the only thing that will take the place of real whipped cream, and it is an effective substitute in some of these desserts. For this reason, choose the best quality topping you can. Cool Whip has never let me down and the light topping is excellent in and on the desserts in this book.

Nonstick cooking spray: Beware! Not all cooking sprays are created equal. Many products on the market fall under this category, but not all give the same results. I specifically recommend unscented, unflavored vegetable oil spray or canola oil spray. These give the best results. Do not be tempted to substitute butter-flavored, olive oil spray, or any diet/lowfat sprays. These will affect the taste of the finished product.

Sour cream: Again, I substitute a light version for regular sour cream, containing 40 calories and 2.5 grams of fat per 2 tablespoons. I have found differences in texture and creaminess from brand to brand, so experiment till you find the one you like best. Read the nutritional information to make sure the calories and fat grams are close to what I have listed above, as some light sour creams have less than others.

Other Ingredients

Almond paste: It is very easy to confuse this with marzipan. For the recipes in this book you will need pure almond paste, which is packed in small rolls or cans. Marzipan is almond paste with sugar added to it, making it ready to use for candy making or cake decorating.

Cherry pie filling: There are many different brands of canned fruit filling on the market, but if you are as choosey as I am, buy the best quality that you can with the most fruit. I find a brand called Comstock to be excellent for the muffin recipe in this book.

Ladyfingers: These crisp Italian sponge biscuits are approximately four inches long and one inch wide. They are perhaps most commonly known for their use in Tiramisù. You can find ladyfingers in gourmet food shops, delicatessens, and food import stores.

Marsala wine: This sweet Italian wine is used in cooking and in making certain Italian desserts. You can find it in liquor stores or in the wine section of your grocery store.

Peanut butter: Many brands are now making a reduced-fat product; however, not all of them are equal in quality. I have found some to be a bit grainy. Use the creamiest one you can find for the best results. I prefer Jif because it really is the creamiest!

Powdered malt: This item can be found in health food stores. I buy it packaged in 8-ounce bags. If you can't find it in powdered form, it is very easy to get in liquid form. It is sold in jars and is usually labeled as malt sweetener or liquid barley malt. Be sure to store the powdered form in a cool, dry place, because high temperatures cause it to break down and become a sticky mess that is no longer usable as a powder.

Sultanas: When you see a recipe asking for sultanas or raisins, it is only a matter of preference. Sultanas are made from white grapes as opposed to the dark purple ones, and have a lighter, fruitier flavor.

Vanilla extract: I feel it is very important to make a stand when it comes to vanilla extract. There is no substitute for pure vanilla extract and the flavor that it imparts to a dessert, so please be sure to always buy pure vanilla instead of imitation. The recipes in this book are depending on it!

Cakes, Tortes, and Tarts

Banana Cream Tart with Brown-Sugar Meringue

Caramel, Pecan, and Banana Cheesecake

Caramel, Pecan, and Coconut Tart

Chocolate Malt Cheesecake

Chocolate Raspberry Sanctuary

Chocolate Whiskey Torte

Classic Cheesecake

Coconut Macaroon Torte

Death by Chocolate

Devil's Food Cake with Fudge Icing

Fresh Berry Tart with Citrus Cream Cheese Filling

Lemon Meringue Cheesecake

Lemon Raspberry Tart

Malted Sponge Cake

Pear Pound Cake

Strawberry Amaretto Shortcakes

Toasted Hazelnut Marble Cheesecake

Tunnel of Peanut Butter Cake

White Chocolate Raspberry Revel

Chapter Three

Cakes, Tortes, and Tarts

If anything exemplifies dessert decadence, it has to be a heavenly slice of cheesecake or a wedge of dark chocolate torte. I can't seem to say no to these delights when the waiter asks, "Would you care for some dessert?" Once those words have been said, it's all over except for the scraping of the plate! It really is difficult for those of us trying so hard to be strong about our diets. Once in a blue moon just isn't often enough when it comes to indulging in chocolate decadence and the like. The memory of each delicious experience only holds the craving off for a day or two before you are craving a luscious dessert again, so much that you would do anything, or say anything, to get your hands on another piece. If I'm hitting too close to home here, then you'll be quite pleased with this chapter. We're talking cakes and tortes and caramel tarts, among other things—just the kind of wicked stuff you would be ordering at your favorite restaurant right about now—all those goodies that make you go "Mmmmmm!!!"

In this chapter you will find everything from simple cakes for afternoon tea or coffee—which can also be elegant after-dinner treasures—to the grandaddy of them all, Death by Chocolate. Then there's everything else in between for any occasion imaginable. Be as creative as you want; Finishing Touches will help you to do just that. Don't take a recipe too literally in its finished form. If you look at a dessert and think, "Hmm, that sure would taste good with some caramel sauce drizzled over it, or a dollop of whipped cream," by all means go right ahead. I have given serving suggestions with the recipes, as this chapter has the most room for experimentation. In the following section you will find some helpful hints for dealing with cakes and tortes.

Pan Preparation

Most of the cake recipes in this book call for lightly coating the pan with nonstick cooking spray and dusting it with flour. By "light coating" I mean there should not be a lot of excess oil to run and drip. I have noticed that some of the sprays bubble when applied. If this happens, simply run your fingers over the surface to smooth out the bubbles before dusting with the flour. I only give this advice for dealing with a cake that will be turned out of the pan, so you don't have to make it all over again because half of it stuck to the bottom of the pan.

Mixing the Batters

In case you missed my General Baking Tips at the beginning of this book, then you should know that I made each of these recipes with a trusty handheld mixer. Most of my cake batters are pretty simple and straightforward, either mixed by hand or with a hand mixer. A few recipes call for beaten egg whites to be folded into the batter. Always fold very gently, and always scrape the bottom and sides of the bowl with a rubber spatula. And when it comes to those batter-covered beaters, it's much wiser to scrape them clean into the bowl rather than into your stomach, as every little bit is crucial to the success of a cake.

Cooling and Inverting

If a cake is to be frosted or covered in velvety ganache, the most important thing to remember is to cool the cake upside down with the smooth side up. This maneuver makes a nice even surface when

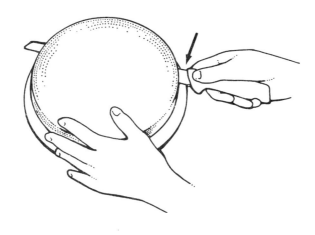

it's time to ice the cake. Many times a cake will end up with a domed top. If it is only a slight dome, don't worry about it. If the dome is significant, however, you can easily level it off with a long serrated knife; otherwise the whole cake will warp if it cools upside down. If you have a cake that needs to have the top preserved—dome or no dome—for a dusting of cocoa or powdered sugar, you will need to invert it twice, using two cake racks. This way the cake will cool right side up, leaving the top unmarked.

Transferring Cakes and Tarts to Serving Platters

It's one thing to bring a dessert to completion, but then you're left wondering how to move that cake or tart to a nice serving platter. This maneuver is much easier than you may think. Just remember, these desserts are not so fragile that the slightest movement will destroy them. If you have read through the equipment descriptions in Chapter Two, you will recall my suggestions for metal icing spatulas and cardboard cake circles. These tools are going to be your best friends in this department!

Tarts are perhaps the easiest of these desserts to transfer from one place to another because you don't have the sides of the pan to contend with. When a tart is completely cool and finished, remove

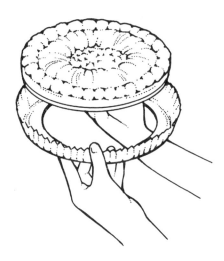

the ring by pushing the whole tart upward from underneath. It will slip right out. Now you have the tart on the metal pan bottom. Slide your angled metal icing spatula between the tart and the metal base, running the tool all along the bottom of the tart to loosen it from the metal. Now that the tart is loose, you can use the spatula to carefully push it onto a plate. Another option is to lift the edge of the loosened tart slightly with the spatula, and slip a cardboard cake circle underneath it. From there you can just leave it on the cake circle or slide it onto another plate.

Much of the same technique applies to cakes. I have found it easiest to handle a cake when it is cold, it is firmer and much more stable for handling. You can transfer a cake by carefully slipping a cardboard cake circle under it. You may find it easier instead to raise the cake's edge slightly with an icing spatula, slide your hand underneath the entire cake, fingers spread wide for support, and simply pick it up and move it as needed. Continue to support the cake using the spatula in your other hand as well. The spatula's low profile will ensure a gentle transition onto the cake's new resting place. You can use the spatula to maneuver the cake around until it's just where you want it, then slide the spatula out with a triumphant flourish.

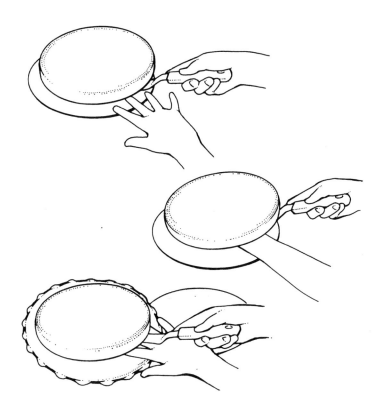

Unmolding and Transferring Cheesecakes

The best way to preserve the condition of your springform pan is to not cut and serve from it. Removing a cheesecake requires a different technique than tarts and cakes. Once the cheesecake has been refrigerated, you can unmold it before adding any final touches or garnishes. Because it has a crumbly graham cracker crust, you cannot move it with a spatula. I have found it very easy to remove a cheesecake from its metal bottom using the following method. However, you won't want to use this method with any cakes that have a topping.

Before unlatching the side ring of the pan, place the whole pan over a burner that has been turned to medium-high heat. Move it

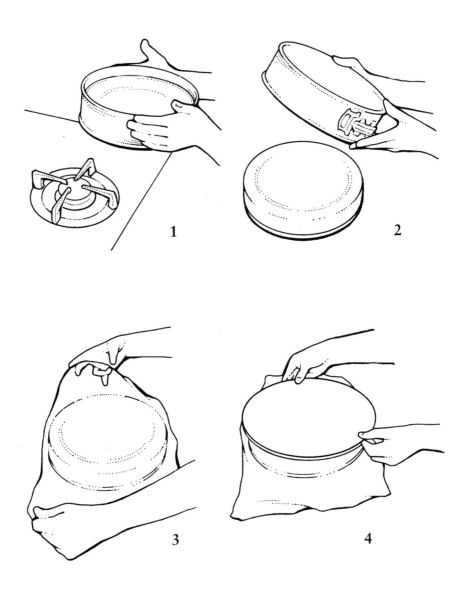

around over the burner for just a few seconds in order to warm the entire bottom of the pan (1). Remove from heat and take off the side ring of the pan (2). Place a sheet of Saran Wrap over the top of the cheesecake (3) and then a cardboard cake circle on top of that (4). Now carefully invert the cheesecake (5). The metal bottom

Sweet Deceptions

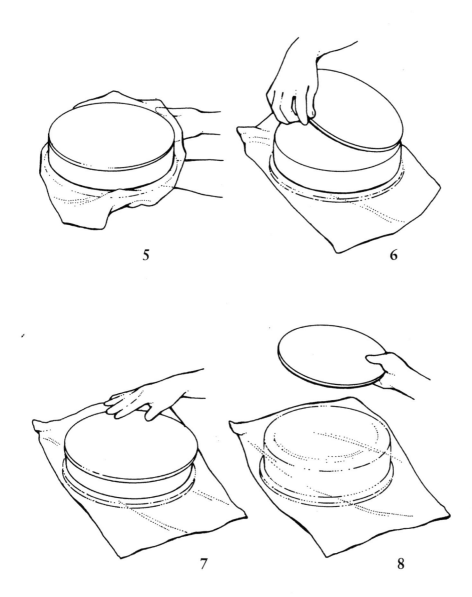

5

6

7

8

should lift right off (6). Place a cardboard cake circle or cake plate over the bottom of the cheesecake and carefully turn it over so that once again it sits right side up (7). Remove the upper cake circle and Saran Wrap (8) and you're ready to add a topping if desired and serve.

Storage

There are some very nice Tupperware-type containers available for keeping whole cakes and tarts airtight. If you don't have such a container, then the best thing you can do is wrap your creations in plastic wrap. When storing a cake that has a frosted or decorated top, stick a few toothpicks into the cake to help keep the wrap from damaging your hard work. Boxes work well too, as long as you push a couple pieces of plastic wrap up against any exposed, cut cake surfaces to keep them from drying out.

Banana Cream Tart with Brown-Sugar Meringue

10 servings

Everyone is familiar with lemon meringue pie, so how about a banana version? This tart is sinfully decadent, with rich banana custard and mounds of unique brown-sugar meringue, crisp on the outside with a fluffy interior.

For crust:

1 1/2 cups all-purpose flour
1/2 cup powdered sugar, sifted
1/4 teaspoon salt
1/4 teaspoon baking powder

1/2 cup (1 stick) light butter, at room temperature
1/4 cup (2 ounces) light Neufchâtel cheese at room temperature

For filling:

1/2 cup liquid nondairy creamer
1/4 cup milk (2 percent)
1 tablespoon cornstarch
1/2 cup granulated sugar

2 large whole eggs plus 2 large egg whites, at room temperature
2 teaspoons vanilla extract
1 medium banana, very ripe

For brown-sugar meringue:

1/4 cup granulated sugar
1/2 cup firmly packed brown sugar

3 large egg whites, at room temperature
1/4 teaspoon cream of tartar

continued

Preheat oven to 350 degrees F. You will need one 9-inch tart pan with removable bottom.

Combine all the crust ingredients to make a soft, pliable dough, using one of three methods. I have found the easiest is in a food processor, fitted with the plastic dough blade. Combine all of the ingredients and process until mixture forms a ball. You can also use a stand mixer with the paddle attachment, mixing all of the ingredients until they form a soft dough or you can combine them by hand.

Place dough on a floured surface and roll out to 1/8-inch thick. Set the tart pan in the center of the dough and trim around it with a sharp knife, leaving a 1 1/2-inch border of dough. You will have excess dough that you can roll out to make a few cookies, or just wrap and freeze it for another use. Slide your hands under the circle of dough and place it in the tart pan. This dough is pliable and easy to work with, without the tendency to crack like pie crust. Press the dough evenly and firmly into all edges of the tart pan. Using a sharp knife, trim off the excess dough flush with the top of the pan. Prick the crust a few times with a toothpick and bake for 15 minutes or until the crust is just beginning to brown. Cool completely on a rack while you prepare the filling.

Keep your oven at 350 degrees F. To make the filling, combine creamer, milk, and cornstarch in a small saucepan. Whisk together until cornstarch has dissolved. Cook over medium heat, stirring with a wooden spoon, until mixture thickens and becomes the consistency of heavy cream. Cool for 10 minutes.

In a medium-size bowl combine sugar, whole eggs, egg whites, and vanilla. Whisk together until smooth. In a food processor combine cooled creamer mixture with banana and process until smooth. Whisk into the egg mixture. Strain custard through a fine-mesh sieve to remove impurities. Pour into prepared crust, still in its pan, and bake for 25 to 30 minutes, until custard is set. Cool completely on a rack, then refrigerate for 1 hour before topping with meringue.

To make the meringue, preheat oven to 375 degrees F. Combine granulated sugar and brown sugar in a food processor and process for approximately 30 seconds to refine the sugar and remove any lumps. In a medium-size mixing bowl (please use stainless steel or glass) that is clean and grease-free, combine the egg whites and cream of tartar. Beat on medium speed of electric mixer until soft peaks form. Increase speed to high and sprinkle in the sugar a tablespoon at a time, beating until all of the sugar has been incorporated and mixture is very stiff and glossy.

This tart has a tendency to produce beads of moisture due to the sugar content in the banana; there may be a syrupy layer on the surface of the custard. You will need to pat it dry before adding the meringue. Gently place a paper towel on the custard surface to absorb the moisture, then carefully lift it off.

Spread the meringue evenly over the surface of the custard, creating any kind of design or swirls that you like. Bake for approximately 10 minutes, or until meringue is light golden brown. Cool completely on a rack, remove it from the pan after it has cooled then refrigerate for at least 1 hour before serving. Store in an airtight container in the refrigerator. Use the hot-knife method described in General Baking Tips to cut this tart.

Serving Suggestions

This dessert is pretty lavish all on its own, but if you really want to go the distance, serve it on a pool of Gooey Caramel Sauce (page 198) and drizzle it with chocolate sauce. However, don't plan on getting up out of your chair for at least a half hour after eating a slice of this beauty!

Each serving provides

246 Calories   22% Calories from Fat   6 g Fat
43 g Carbohydrates   5 g Protein   31 mg Calcium
1 g Dietary Fiber   168 mg Sodium   55 mg Cholesterol

Caramel, Pecan, and Banana Cheesecake

16 servings

This creation was one of my most popular cheesecakes in its fattening form, so I knew I had to find a way to incorporate it into this book. It turned out to be easier than I thought. Not only did I lower the calories and fat, I managed to maintain its sinful texture of creamy banana cheesecake with swirls of gooey caramel and toasted pecans. Don't be surprised to find yourself hiding pieces of it because you can't bear to share!

For crust:

3   whole graham crackers, finely crushed

1/2 cup plain dry bread crumbs

1/4 teaspoon ground allspice

1 1/2 tablespoons light butter, melted

For caramel pecan swirl:

1/2 cup Gooey Caramel Sauce (page 198)

1 1/2 ounces (approximately 1/2 cup) crushed (not ground) toasted pecans

For filling:

1   cup lowfat cottage cheese

1/3 cup brown sugar, firmly packed

1   tablespoon vanilla extract

1   medium banana, very ripe

1   cup (8 ounces) light Neufchâtel cheese, at room temperature

1 1/2 cups (12 ounces) fat-free cream cheese, at room temperature

1/3 cup granulated sugar

2   whole large eggs, at room temperature

1   large egg white, at room temperature

2   large egg whites, at room temperature

2   tablespoons granulated sugar

Preheat oven to 350 degrees F. Lightly coat the bottom of an 8-inch or 9-inch springform pan with nonstick cooking spray.

Combine all the crust ingredients, using your hands to coat the crumbs with the butter to make a uniform mixture. Press evenly and firmly over the bottom of prepared pan. Bake for 10 to 15 minutes, until crust is light golden brown and crisp. Set aside to cool.

To make the swirl, combine the pecans with the caramel and set aside at room temperature until ready to use.

To make the filling, preheat oven to 325 degrees F. In a food processor fitted with the metal blade puree cottage cheese, brown sugar, vanilla, and banana. Process until smooth. In a large mixing bowl combine Neufchâtel cheese, cream cheese, and the 1/3 cup granulated sugar. Cream on medium speed of electric mixer until smooth. Beat in the cottage cheese mixture, then the 2 whole eggs and 1 egg white just until incorporated and batter is smooth.

In a medium-size mixing bowl that is clean and grease-free, beat the remaining 2 egg whites on medium speed of electric mixer until soft peaks form. Increase speed to high and sprinkle in the remaining 2 tablespoons of sugar and continue beating until firm peaks form. Carefully fold the beaten egg whites into the batter, using a rubber spatula. Batter should be uniform, with no streaks of egg white showing.

Pour half the batter into prepared pan and smooth the top. Dot the surface with half of the caramel-pecan mixture and swirl it into the batter with an icing spatula or a knife. Do not completely blend it in; it should look marbled and swirled.

Pour the remaining batter into the pan and repeat the swirling process with the rest of the caramel-pecan mixture.

Bake for 50 minutes to 1 hour. Cake will be springy when lightly touched in the center and slightly cracked around the edges,

continued

Cakes, Tortes, and Tarts

due to its lightness. Turn off the oven and allow cake to cool for one hour with the oven door ajar. Finish cooling on a rack at room temperature, then refrigerate for at least 6 hours or overnight before removing from pan and cutting, using the hot-knife method described in General Baking Tips.

Serving Suggestions

Try a dollop of light whipped topping, or drizzle a slice with extra Gooey Caramel Sauce (page 198). You can also serve it on a pool of Crème Anglaise (page 197) splashed with caramel and chocolate sauces.

Each serving provides

208 Calories   30% Calories from Fat   7 g Fat
27 g Carbohydrates   9 g Protein   117 mg Calcium
9 g Dietary Fiber   363 mg Sodium   45 mg Cholesterol

Caramel, Pecan, and Coconut Tart

12 servings

I can never seem to turn down a piece of pecan pie, regardless of its calorie and fat content, which would throw the needle completely off the meter and straight to Mars! Since it's the flavor that is so addictive, I just did away with most of the pecans, which were the major fat culprit, and filled in with coconut. This tart is a wonderful substitute for pecan pie as I have kept all of the familiar flavors intact, wrapped up in a caramel custard with flaked coconut and an acceptable amount of pecans.

For crust:

1 1/2 cups all-purpose flour

1/2 cup powdered sugar, sifted

1/4 teaspoon salt

1/4 teaspoon baking powder

1/2 cup (1 stick) light butter at room temperature

1/4 cup (2 ounces) light Neufchâtel cheese, at room temperature

For filling:

3/4 cup firmly packed brown sugar

1/2 cup light corn syrup

1/2 cup dark corn syrup

3 large egg whites, at room temperature

1/2 teaspoon salt

1 tablespoon vanilla extract

2 teaspoons butter-flavored extract

2 tablespoons all-purpose flour

1/2 teaspoon ground allspice

3/4 cup toasted, sweetened, flaked coconut

1/3 cup toasted, chopped pecans

continued

Preheat oven to 350 degrees F. You will need one 9-inch tart pan with removable bottom.

Combine all the crust ingredients to make a soft, pliable dough, using one of three methods. I have found the easiest is in a food processor, fitted with the plastic dough blade. Combine all of the ingredients and process until the mixture forms a ball. You can also use a stand mixer with the paddle attachment, mixing all of the ingredients until they form a soft dough. As a last resort, you can combine them by hand.

Place dough on a floured surface and roll out to 1/8-inch thick. Set the tart pan in the center of the dough and trim around it with a sharp knife, leaving a 1 1/2-inch border of dough. Reserve the excess dough for optional decorative cutouts for the top of the tart. Slide your hands under the circle of dough and place it in the tart pan. This dough is pliable and easy to work with, and does not have the tendency to crack like pie crust. Press the dough evenly and firmly into all edges of the tart pan. Use a sharp knife to trim off the excess dough flush with the top of the pan. Set aside to prepare filling.

For optional decorations, roll out remaining dough and cut into any desired shape, no larger than 1 1/2 inches squared. I like to cut out small hearts. Place on a cookie sheet lined with foil or parchment paper and bake at 350 degrees F for 10 to 15 minutes, until they are light golden brown.

To make the filling, in a medium-size bowl combine brown sugar, both corn syrups, egg whites, salt, vanilla, and butter extract. Whisk together until smooth. Whisk in the flour and allspice. Stir in the coconut and pecans. Pour filling into prepared crust and bake for 30 to 35 minutes, until filling is set and no longer liquid. Cool completely on a rack before removing from pan, then cut into 12 pieces using the hot-knife method described in General Baking Tips. Store wrapped in plastic or in an airtight container in the refrigerator. Serve at room temperature. To decorate with pastry cutouts, after cutting the tart place a cutout on each slice, securing it with a dab of corn syrup.

Sweet Deceptions

Serving Suggestions

This tart is at its absolute best on a pool of Gem Caramel Sauce (page 200) with a dollop of light whipped topping. Don't forget a sprig of mint!

I have also found that Chocolate Ganache (page 206) makes a nice accompaniment. Warm the ganache and drizzle it all across the top of tart, in place of the cutouts. If you don't care for whipped topping, try the Crème Anglaise (page 197) or A la Mode (page 190) with a scoop of frozen yogurt.

Each serving provides

309 Calories   26% Calories from Fat   9 g Fat
56 g Carbohydrates   4 g Protein   23 mg Calcium
1 g Dietary Fiber   273 mg Sodium   17 mg Cholesterol

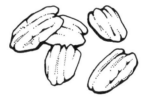

Cakes, Tortes, and Tarts

Chocolate Malt Cheesecake

If you ever had a true chocolate malt, then you will fully appreciate the distinctive and wonderful flavor of this cheesecake. Malt sweetener gives this cheesecake its unique taste, a bit reminiscent of malted milk candy.

For crust:

3 whole graham crackers, finely crushed

1/2 cup plain dry bread crumbs

1 1/2 tablespoons light butter, melted

For filling:

1 cup lowfat small-curd cottage cheese

1 1/2 cup (12 ounces) fat-free cream cheese, at room temperature

1 tablespoon vanilla extract

3/4 cup granulated sugar

12 ounces light Neufchâtel cheese, at room temperature

1/2 cup unsweetened cocoa, sifted

1/2 cup powdered malt (or 1/4 cup liquid barley malt)

1 large whole egg, at room temperature

2 large egg whites, at room temperature

2 large egg whites, at room temperature

2 tablespoons granulated sugar

Preheat oven to 350 degrees F. Lightly coat the bottom of an 8-inch or 9-inch springform pan with vegetable or canola oil spray. Combine all the crust ingredients, using your hands to coat the crumbs with butter to make a uniform mixture. Press evenly and firmly over the bottom of prepared pan. Bake for 10 to 15 minutes, until crust is light golden brown and crisp. Set aside to cool.

To make the filling, preheat oven to 325 degrees F. In a food processor fitted with the metal blade, puree the cottage cheese, cream cheese, and vanilla. Process until smooth and creamy.

In a large mixing bowl cream the 3/4 cup sugar and Neufchâtel cheese on medium speed of electric mixer until smooth. Blend in cottage cheese mixture. Add cocoa and malt. Reduce speed to low and beat until fully incorporated. Add the whole egg and 2 egg whites, beating just until they are combined.

In a separate medium-size mixing bowl that is clean and grease-free, beat the remaining 2 egg whites on medium speed of electric mixer until soft peaks form. Increase speed to high and sprinkle in the remaining 2 tablespoons of sugar, a tablespoon at a time, beating until firm peaks form. Carefully fold the beaten egg whites into the batter using a rubber spatula. Batter should be uniform, with no streaks of egg white showing. Pour into prepared pan and smooth the top with a rubber spatula.

Bake for 50 minutes to 1 hour. Cake will be springy when lightly touched in the center, and slightly cracked around the edges due to its lightness. Turn off the oven and allow cake to cool for one hour with the oven door ajar. Finish cooling at room temperature, then refrigerate for at least 6 hours or overnight before removing from pan and cutting into 16 pieces using the hot-knife method described in General Baking Tips. Store in an airtight container in the refrigerator.

Serving Suggestions

Try this cheesecake on a pool of Gooey Caramel Sauce (page 198). You can also serve it on a custard sauce (page 197), or with a dollop of Light Whipped Topping (page 189). If you want to decorate it, try finishing it with Chocolate Ganache (page 206) and Crushed Meringue (page 208) dusted with cocoa or powdered sugar.

Each serving provides

190 Calories   32% Calories from Fat   7 g Fat
23 g Carbohydrates   10 g Protein   111 mg Calcium
0 g Dietary Fiber   340 mg Sodium   36 mg Cholesterol

Chocolate Raspberry Sanctuary

12 servings

Here you will find sweet refuge from the everyday rat race. Just lose yourself in a sanctuary of sweet ripe raspberries floating in chocolate ganache, atop an intense chocolate brownie cake.

For cake:

3 ounces (3 squares) unsweetened chocolate

2 tablespoons brewed black coffee

1/4 cup plus 1 tablespoon dark corn syrup

3/4 cup all-purpose flour

1/4 teaspoon baking soda

3/4 teaspoon salt

3/4 cup granulated sugar

1 large whole egg plus 1 large egg white, at room temperature

1/3 cup fat-free ricotta cheese

1 tablespoon vanilla extract

For ganache:

1/3 cup (1 1/2 ounces) semi-sweet chocolate chips

2 tablespoons liquid nondairy creamer

For assembly:

1 3/4 cups fresh raspberries

Preheat oven to 350 degrees F. Lightly coat an 8 × 2-inch round cake pan with vegetable or canola oil spray and dust with flour. In a small saucepan combine chocolate, coffee, and all the corn syrup. Melt over low heat, stirring until smooth. Remove from heat and cool for 10 minutes.

In a small bowl combine flour, baking soda, and salt. In a medium-size bowl combine sugar, whole egg, egg white, ricotta, and vanilla. Whisk together until smooth. Whisk in cooled chocolate mixture. Stir in dry ingredients to make a smooth batter. Pour into prepared pan and dot the raspberry jam over the batter, using

Sweet Deceptions

a knife or toothpick to swirl it around, giving the surface a marbled look.

Bake for 18 to 20 minutes. Cake should indent slightly when touched in center; do not bake for longer than 20 minutes. Cake is intended to be very moist and fudgy. Cool cake in pan for 2 to 3 minutes, then turn it out onto a cake rack. Use a second rack to invert again so the cake cools right side up.

To make the ganache, in a small non-metallic bowl combine chocolate chips and liquid creamer. Microwave on medium-high for 30 to 60 seconds, just until chocolate is melted. For stovetop use, combine ingredients in a small saucepan and melt over low heat. Stir until smooth.

For final assembly, spread the ganache evenly over the top of cake using an icing spatula. Neatly arrange the raspberries on top of the ganache to cover the entire surface. Working from the outside edge toward the center is best. Cut cake into 12 servings, using the hot-knife method described in General Baking Tips.

This cake should be kept in an airtight container in the refrigerator and served by the next day, due to the fresh raspberries. However, it will taste best if brought to room temperature before serving.

Serving Suggestions

There aren't many things that can compare to the combined flavors of chocolate and fresh raspberries. It would seem only fitting to bathe a piece of this wonderful torte in a gem-like pool of Raspberry Sauce (page 202). This is my favorite way to serve it. You can also serve it with a dollop of light whipped topping. For the ultimate chocolate experience, try serving it on a pool of Chocolate Sauce (page 201).

Each serving provides

197 Calories   28% Calories from Fat   6 g Fat
35 g Carbohydrates   4 g Protein   36 mg Calcium
1 g Dietary Fiber   192 mg Sodium   18 mg Cholesterol

Chocolate Whiskey Torte

12 servings

If you want this torte to be truly at its best, get ahold of a bottle of Gentleman Jack Tennessee Whiskey. I borrowed a bit of my husband's supply one day when he wasn't looking, because it was the only whiskey we had in the house. Now I've been spoiled and have to use it every time I make this torte! You can, however, use any quality brand whiskey you like and end up with a delicious cake.

For cake:

1 ounce (1 square) unsweetened chocolate	3/4 cup lowfat, small-curd cottage cheese
1/4 cup dark corn syrup	1 cup granulated sugar
1 tablespoon water	2 teaspoons vanilla extract
1 cup all-purpose flour	3 large egg whites, at room temperature
1/2 cup unsweetened cocoa	1/4 cup whiskey, plus 1 1/2 tablespoons to brush on cake
1 1/2 teaspoons baking powder	
3/4 teaspoon salt	
1/4 cup (1/2 stick) light butter at room temperature	

For ganache filling:

1/3 cup (1 1/2 ounces) semisweet chocolate chips	2 tablespoons liquid nondairy creamer

For assembly:

2 tablespoons powdered sugar, approximately

Preheat oven to 350 degrees F. Lightly coat two 8 × 2-inch round baking pans with vegetable or canola oil spray and dust with flour.

In a small saucepan combine chocolate, corn syrup, and water. Place over low heat and melt until smooth, stirring occasionally. Set aside to cool.

In a small bowl combine flour, cocoa, baking powder, and salt. In a food processor fitted with the metal blade, cream the butter, cottage cheese, sugar, and vanilla. Process for 30 seconds, until mixture is smooth. Add egg whites and process until they are incorporated.

Pour mixture into a large mixing bowl and whisk in the cooled chocolate mixture along with the 1/4 cup whiskey. Whisk in the flour mixture by hand or on low speed of electric mixer, just until batter is uniform and smooth. Divide batter evenly between prepared pans and smooth with a spatula.

Bake for 18 to 20 minutes, or until cake tester inserted into the center comes out clean. (A few moist crumbs on it are okay.) Cool in pans for 2 to 3 minutes before turning them out onto a cake rack to cool completely.

To make the ganache, in a small non-metallic bowl combine chocolate chips and liquid creamer. Microwave on medium-high for 30 to 60 seconds, just until chocolate is melted. For stovetop use, combine the ingredients in a small saucepan and melt over low heat. Stir mixture until smooth.

To assemble the cake, brush the bottom cake layer with the remaining 1 1/2 tablespoons of whiskey, using a pastry brush. With an icing spatula, spread the ganache filling evenly over cake layer. Top with second cake. Dust cake with powdered sugar, sifting it through a fine-mesh sieve. Cut into 12 pieces using the hot-knife method described in General Baking Tips. Store cake in an airtight container in the refrigerator, and bring to room temperature before serving.

Serving Suggestions

I like to put dark chocolate curls around the edge of the cake before dusting with the powdered sugar, and then sift the sugar over the chocolate curls. This extra effort makes a really elegant torte. Add a dollop of light whipped topping and you're all set.

You can also serve it on Crème Anglaise (page 197) splashed with Chocolate Sauce (page 201)—maybe even some caramel sauce for a triple decadent effect.

Each serving provides

209 Calories   26% Calories from Fat   6 g Fat
35 g Carbohydrates   5 g Protein   22 mg Calcium
1 g Dietary Fiber   253 mg Sodium   7 mg Cholesterol

Classic Cheesecake

12 servings

This cheesecake is the purest: no frills, fillings, or toppings, and a lot less fat and calories. You'll find it a little lighter than traditional cheesecake, but you won't be missing out on any of the traditional flavor.

For crust:

3 whole graham crackers, finely crushed

1/2 cup plain dry bread crumbs

1/4 teaspoon ground cinnamon

1 1/2 tablespoons light butter, melted

For filling:

2 cups (16 ounces) light Neufchâtel cheese at room temperature

1 1/2 cups (12 ounces) fat-free cream cheese, at room temperature

3/4 cup granulated sugar

2 large whole eggs, at room temperature

1 tablespoon vanilla extract

3 large egg whites, at room temperature

1 tablespoon granulated sugar

Preheat oven to 350 degrees F. Lightly coat the bottom of an 8-inch or 9-inch springform pan with vegetable or canola oil spray.

Combine all the crust ingredients, using your hands to coat the crumbs with the butter to make a uniform mixture. Press evenly and firmly into the bottom of prepared pan. Bake for 10 to 15 minutes, until crust is light golden brown and crisp. Set aside to cool while you make the filling.

Lower oven temperature to 325 degrees F. In a large mixing bowl cream Neufchâtel cheese, cream cheese, and the 3/4 cup sugar on medium speed of electric mixer until smooth. Add whole eggs and vanilla, mixing just until eggs are incorporated and batter is smooth.

In a medium-size mixing bowl that is clean and grease-free, beat the egg whites on medium speed of electric mixer until soft peaks form. Increase speed to high and sprinkle in remaining tablespoon of sugar, beating until firm peaks form. Carefully fold the beaten egg whites into the batter using a rubber spatula. Batter should be uniform, with no streaks of egg white showing. Pour into prepared pan and smooth the top.

Bake for 50 minutes to 1 hour. Cake will be springy when lightly touched in the center, and slightly cracked around the edges due to its lightness. Turn off the oven and allow cake to cool for one hour with the oven door ajar. Finish cooling on a rack at room temperature, then refrigerate for at least 6 hours or overnight before removing from pan and cutting into 12 pieces using the hot-knife method described in General Baking Tips. Store in an airtight container in the refrigerator.

Serving Suggestions

Anything goes with this one. Because of this cheesecake's simple, elegant flavor, you can serve it with just about anything you can imagine, from fresh berries and berry purees to caramel sauce. The fruit, however, does seem to complement it the best.

Each serving provides

229 Calories   43% Calories from Fat   11 g Fat
21 g Carbohydrates   11 g Protein   139 mg Calcium
0 g Dietary Fiber   412 mg Sodium   73 mg Cholesterol

Coconut Macaroon Torte

16 servings

Attention all coconut fans! Here's the cake that you've been dreaming about: A moist, lightly scented coconut cake perched atop a chewy coconut macaroon layer and then covered in rich dark chocolate.

For coconut macaroon base:

- 3 large egg whites, at room temperature
- 3/4 cup powdered sugar
- 2 tablespoons light corn syrup
- 2 teaspoons vanilla extract
- 1/2 cup all-purpose flour
- 2 cups flaked, sweetened coconut

For cake:

- 3/4 cup milk (2 percent)
- 1/2 cup sweetened, flaked coconut
- 1 1/2 cups all-purpose flour
- 2 teaspoons baking powder
- 1/2 teaspoon salt
- 3/4 cup granulated sugar
- 2 tablespoons vegetable shortening
- 1/4 cup lowfat ricotta cheese
- 1 large egg white, at room temperature
- 2 teaspoons vanilla extract

- 2 large egg whites, at room temperature
- 2 tablespoons granulated sugar

For dark chocolate glaze:

- 4 tablespoons liquid nondairy creamer
- 1/2 cup semisweet chocolate chips
- 1 square unsweetened chocolate, chopped

Lightly coat a 10-inch springform pan with vegetable or canola oil spray and dust with flour. To make macaroon base, in a medium-size bowl combine egg whites, sugar, corn syrup, and vanilla. Whisk together until smooth and creamy. Whisk in the flour until fully incorporated. Stir in coconut. Spread mixture evenly on the bottom of prepared springform pan, using a rubber spatula. Set aside while you make the cake.

Preheat oven to 350 degrees F. In a small saucepan combine milk and coconut. Cook over medium-high heat until mixture begins to simmer. Remove from heat and cool completely. Strain milk through a fine-mesh sieve, pressing out all of the liquid from the coconut. Discard coconut.

In a small bowl combine flour, baking powder, and salt. In a medium-size bowl combine sugar, shortening, and ricotta, and beat on medium speed of electric mixer until creamy. Add flour alternately with the cooled coconut milk, beating after each addition until the batter is smooth. Beat in 1 egg white and vanilla until fully incorporated.

In a small mixing bowl that is clean and grease-free, beat the remaining 2 egg whites on medium speed of electric mixer until soft peaks form. Increase speed to high and sprinkle in the sugar a tablespoon at a time, beating until firm peaks form. Stir a third of the egg whites into the batter to loosen it up, then carefully fold in the remaining beaten egg whites with a rubber spatula. Pour batter into prepared springform pan, over the macaroon base.

Bake for 40 to 50 minutes, or until a cake tester inserted into the center comes out clean. Cool completely on a rack, in pan. When cake is cool, transfer to a plate or cake circle using the inverting method for cheesecakes (see tips at the beginning of this chapter).

To make the glaze, in a small saucepan heat the creamer over high heat until it reaches a boil. Remove from heat and add all the chocolate. Let stand for a couple of minutes before stirring until smooth. If chocolate has not melted completely, you may return it to the stove over medium heat, and stir until melted and smooth.

continued

To finish the cake, pour glaze over cooled cake, coaxing it down the sides. You can use an icing spatula to spread icing over entire top and sides of cake, or you can just let the icing drip down. Let glaze cool for at least half an hour before cutting the cake. If you need to transfer the cake to another plate or serving platter, see the hints at the beginning of this chapter. Store in an airtight container in the refrigerator, but cake tastes best when served at room temperature.

Serving Suggestions

Be sure to sprinkle some toasted coconut over the top of the cake. There are all kinds of ways you could serve this dessert, but my favorite would have to be presenting it on a pool of Gooey Caramel Sauce (page 198) with a few toasted nuts—then you really feel like you're eating a candy bar! Also, try Raspberry Sauce (page 202) and Chocolate Curls (page 191).

Each serving provides

267 Calories   35% Calories from Fat   11 g Fat
40 g Carbohydrates   5 g Protein   50 mg Calcium
2 g Dietary Fiber   180 mg Sodium   2 mg Cholesterol

Death by Chocolate

20 servings

Only deeply committed, self-confessed chocoholics who live for the rush that can only come from unrestrained chocolate consumption should even dare to look twice at this recipe. This is serious chocolate: layers of chocolate in all different forms, from crisp chocolate meringue and real chocolate buttercream to dense and intense chocolate cake and rich dark chocolate ganache. This is a big cake and it means business! It's the perfect dessert to make for your next birthday or dinner party. The meringue layers can be made up to a week in advance provided they are stored in an airtight container. The cake layers can be made up to one day in advance. The ganache and frosting can also be made two to three days ahead if stored in airtight containers in the refrigerator.

For crisp chocolate meringue layers:

- 3 large egg whites, at room temperature
- 1/4 teaspoon cream of tartar
- 3/4 cup granulated sugar
- 1/4 cup unsweetened cocoa, sifted

For chocolate brownie cake layers:

- 5 ounces (5 squares) unsweetened chocolate
- 1 1/4 cup plus 2 tablespoons dark corn syrup
- 2 1/2 tablespoons canola oil
- 1 3/4 cup plus 2 tablespoons all-purpose flour
- 3/4 teaspoon baking soda
- 1 1/2 teaspoons salt
- 1/2 cup plus 2 tablespoons fat-free ricotta cheese
- 1/2 cup plus 2 tablespoons granulated sugar
- 2 large whole eggs, at room temperature
- 3 large egg whites, at room temperature
- 2 1/2 tablespoons vanilla extract

continued

For chocolate ganache:

1/3 cup plus 1 tablespoon liquid nondairy creamer	1 1/2 cups semisweet chocolate chips

For chocolate buttercream frosting:

3/4 cup granulated sugar	3/4 cup (1 1/2 sticks) unsalted butter, at room temperature
1/4 teaspoon salt	
1/3 cup water	
1/3 cup (approximately 3 large) egg whites, at room temperature	1/4 cup butter-flavored shortening
	1 teaspoon vanilla extract
1/4 teaspoon cream of tartar	6 tablespoons unsweetened cocoa, sifted
2 tablespoons granulated sugar	

Preheat oven to its lowest setting, which should be less than 200 degrees F. You will need 2 cookie sheets lined with parchment paper or foil. Trace one 8-inch circle on each cookie sheet. Set aside to prepare meringue.

In a medium-size mixing bowl that is clean and grease-free, combine egg whites and cream of tartar. Beat on medium speed of electric mixer until soft peaks form. Increase speed to high and sprinkle in the sugar, a tablespoon at a time, beating until all of the sugar has been incorporated and meringue is very stiff and glossy. Carefully fold in the sifted cocoa in two additions, using a rubber spatula, until cocoa is incorporated.

Divide meringue evenly between the two cookie sheets. Use an icing spatula to spread the meringue all the way to the edges of the circles, as levelly as possible. Don't worry about them being perfect because you can trim the edges after they have baked.

Place meringue discs in warm oven to dry out overnight. This slow baking preserves the meringues' delicate structure, making them crunchy and light in texture. When meringues are crisp, remove from oven and cool for 15 minutes. Carefully peel the meringues off the paper or foil and store in an airtight container

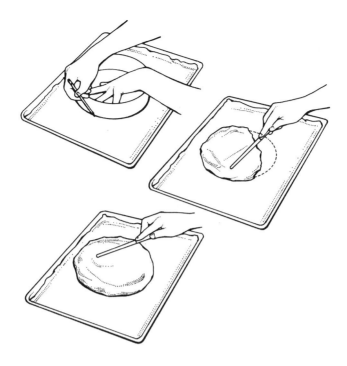

until ready to assemble cake. A large Ziploc bag works best for this. The meringues are fragile, so handle them gently. If you do happen to break one, don't worry. You can piece it back together when you assemble the cake.

To make the cake, preheat oven to 350 degrees F. Lightly coat three 8 × 2-inch round baking pans with vegetable or canola oil spray and dust with flour.

In a medium-size saucepan combine chocolate, all the corn syrup, and oil. Melt over low heat, stirring until smooth. Remove from heat and cool for ten minutes.

In a small bowl stir together flour, baking soda, and salt. In a large bowl combine ricotta, all the sugar, whole eggs, egg whites, and vanilla. Whisk together until smooth. Whisk in cooled chocolate mixture. Stir in dry ingredients to make a smooth batter. Divide evenly among the prepared pans.

continued

Cakes, Tortes, and Tarts   51

Bake for 17 to 20 minutes. Cake should indent slightly when touched in the center. Turn cakes out onto racks to cool completely. Store in airtight containers until ready to assemble dessert.

To make the ganache, in a small saucepan heat the creamer over high heat until it reaches a boil. Remove from heat and add the chocolate chips. Let stand for a couple of minutes before stirring until smooth. If chocolate has not melted completely, you may return it to the stove over medium heat and stir until melted and smooth. Cool completely and store in an airtight container in the refrigerator until ready to assemble cake. Bring to room temperature before use.

To make the buttercream, in a small saucepan combine the 3/4 cup sugar, salt, and water. Place over high heat and clip a candy thermometer onto the pan. Cook the sugar, undisturbed, until it reaches the soft ball stage on the thermometer, which is 240 degrees F. Meanwhile, combine the egg whites and cream of tartar in a medium-size mixing bowl. When the sugar syrup reaches about 220 degrees F, begin beating the egg whites on medium speed of electric mixer until soft peaks form. Increase speed to high and sprinkle in the remaining 2 tablespoons sugar, a tablespoon at a time, beating until firm peaks form.

By now the sugar syrup should be at the proper temperature. Pour the hot syrup into the egg whites in a slow, steady stream while beating on high speed. Move the beaters around the bowl to evenly distribute the syrup if you're using a hand mixer. Continue to beat until meringue is room temperature to the touch, and stands stiff and glossy.

At this point, slow the mixer to medium speed and add the butter and shortening all at once. Once they have been incorporated, increase speed to high again and continue to beat until icing is fluffy. It is important that the egg whites not be warm when you add the butter, or the icing will become curdled and soupy, due to the melting of the butter. If this does happen, you can still save the batch of icing as long as it is only slightly soupy and not a full-blown curdled mess! Simply beat in a little more butter or shortening, until the icing comes together and firms up. This may change your calorie and fat counts a bit, but it's better than starting all over again.

Store in an airtight container in the refrigerator until ready to assemble cake. Icing must be at room temperature to use.

Before you begin to assemble this small monument, make sure you have all of the elements, and that the ganache and buttercream are at room temperature and of spreading consistency. Choose a nice flat serving plate for the foundation. Make sure all three cake layers are level without domed tops; you can use a serrated knife to trim them if you need to.

Place one cake layer on the plate and spread the top of it with half of the chocolate ganache. Now top with one of the chocolate meringue disks. If the disc looks too large in circumference, simply trim it down with a serrated knife. Spread the meringue disk with one third of the chocolate buttercream and top with the second cake layer.

Repeat these steps to finish building the cake—ganache, meringue, buttercream, cake. The top of the cake will be covered with the last third of the buttercream. This is supposed to be a rustic-looking cake with all of its layers exposed. For the grand finale, you can top it with dark chocolate and white chocolate curls and then dust them with cocoa, using a fine-mesh sieve. This is a showy cake, and is very impressive when sliced, as the slices seem larger than life!

Refrigerating this dessert for an hour will make cutting it a bit easier; use the hot-knife method described in General Baking Tips. If you prefer, cut it at room temperature with a sharp knife. Store cake in an airtight container in the refrigerator, but serve at room temperature.

Serving Suggestions

This is uncharted territory and I'm not about to go exploring! If you feel you can handle anything being added to this dessert, take your pick from Finishing Touches.

Each serving provides

425 Calories   45% Calories from Fat   22 g Fat
59 g Carbohydrates   6 g Protein   41 mg Calcium
1 g Dietary Fiber   321 mg Sodium   42 mg Cholesterol

Devil's Food Cake with Fudge Icing

20 servings

This cake is devilishly chocolaty, and about as close to the real thing as you can get! I make this one big—two layers tall and ten inches across—and serve it for birthday parties.

For cake:

3 cups all-purpose flour
3/4 cup unsweetened cocoa
1 tablespoon baking powder
2 teaspoons baking soda
1 teaspoon salt
1 cup brown sugar, firmly packed
1/2 cup granulated sugar

1/4 cup canola oil
1/2 cup lowfat ricotta cheese
4 large egg whites, at room temperature
1 1/2 tablespoons vanilla extract
1/4 cup cider vinegar
1 3/4 cup milk (2 percent)

For fudge icing:

1/3 cup liquid non-dairy creamer
1/2 cup semisweet chocolate chips
2 ounces (2 squares) unsweetened baking chocolate

1/2 teaspoon salt
1 tablespoon light butter
2 teaspoons vanilla extract
2 cups powdered sugar, sifted

Preheat oven to 350 degrees F. Generously coat two 10 × 2-inch round cake pans with vegetable or canola oil spray and dust with flour. In a large mixing bowl, combine flour, cocoa, baking powder, baking soda, and salt. In a separate mixing bowl, combine brown sugar, granulated sugar, canola oil, and ricotta. Beat with electric mixer on medium speed until creamy and smooth. Beat in egg whites and vanilla until fully incorporated, then beat in vinegar. Pour batter into dry ingredients along with the milk. Beat with an electric mixer on medium speed until smooth and creamy. Divide batter evenly between the prepared pans and bake 25 to 35 minutes or until a cake tester inserted into the center comes out clean. Immediately invert cakes onto wire cooling racks and cool completely before assembling and icing cake.

To make the icing, combine creamer, chocolate chips, unsweetened chocolate, salt, and light butter in a small saucepan. Place over medium heat and stir until melted and smooth. Remove from heat and transfer mixture to a medium-size mixing bowl. Beat in vanilla and powdered sugar, 1/2 cup at a time, on medium speed of electric mixer until all the sugar has been incorporated and icing is smooth and creamy. Transfer first cake layer to a plate or serving platter and spread the top with half the icing. Place second layer on top of the first and cover with the remaining icing. Let cake stand for at least 30 minutes to set the icing. Cut into 20 slices using the hot-knife method described in General Baking Tips and serve at room temperature. Store cake loosely wrapped with plastic in the refrigerator.

Serving Suggestions

This particular cake happens to be the one I'm balancing on my finger on the cover of this book. The only other thing I like to do with it is top it with milk chocolate curls for a decadent finale!

Each serving provides

273 Calories   27% Calories from Fat   8 g Fat
47 g Carbohydrates   5 g Protein   88 mg Calcium
1 g Dietary Fiber   359 mg Sodium   5 mg Cholesterol

Fresh Berry Tart with Citrus Cream Cheese Filling

Take a walk on the lighter side with this refreshing berry tart. You may use any kind of fresh berry, but I prefer to use a combination for the contrast of flavors and textures.

For crust:

1½ cups all-purpose flour

½ cup powdered sugar, sifted

¼ teaspoon salt

¼ teaspoon baking powder

½ cup (1 stick) light butter, at room temperature

¼ cup (2 ounces) light Neufchâtel cheese, at room temperature

For citrus cream cheese filling:

½ cup (4 ounces) fat-free cream cheese at room temperature

½ cup (4 ounces) light Neufchâtel cheese, at room temperature

½ cup powdered sugar

1 teaspoon vanilla extract

½ teaspoon lemon extract

2 teaspoons grated lemon peel

2 teaspoons grated lime peel

2 teaspoons grated orange peel

1 large egg white, at room temperature

1½ tablespoons granulated sugar

For assembly:

Approximately 4 cups fresh berries

Preheat oven to 350 degrees F. You will need one 9-inch tart pan with removable bottom. Combine all the crust ingredients to make a soft, pliable dough using one of three methods. I have found the easiest is in a food processor, fitted with the plastic dough blade, combining all of the ingredients and processing until mixture forms a ball. You can also use a stand mixer with the paddle attachment, mixing all of the ingredients until they form a soft dough. As a last resort, you can combine them by hand.

Place dough on a floured surface and roll out to 1/8-inch thick. Set the tart pan in the center of the dough and trim around it with a sharp knife leaving a 1 1/2-inch border of dough. You will have excess dough that you can roll out to make a few cookies, or just wrap and freeze it for another use. Slide your hands under the circle of dough and place it in the tart pan. This dough is pliable and easy to work with, and does not have the tendency to crack like pie crust. Press the dough evenly and firmly into all edges of the tart pan. Use a sharp knife to trim off the excess dough, flush with the top of the pan. Prick crust a few times with a toothpick and bake for 15 to 20 minutes, until crust is light golden brown. Cool completely on a rack while you prepare the filling.

In a small mixing bowl combine both cream cheeses, powdered sugar, vanilla, lemon extract, and all three grated peels. Beat on medium speed of electric mixer until smooth and creamy.

In a separate small mixing bowl that is clean and grease-free, beat the egg white on medium speed of electric mixer until soft peaks form. Sprinkle in the granulated sugar and continue beating until firm peaks form. Carefully fold beaten egg white into sweet cheese mixture, and spread evenly into tart shell. Refrigerate for 1 hour before topping with berries.

The exact amount of each berry you will need for the final assembly depends on how you plan to arrange them on the tart. I usually use 1 1/2 cups of blackberries around the outside, then 3/4 to 1 cup of raspberries, and 3/4 cup of blueberries in the center. The

continued

Cakes, Tortes, and Tarts

combination of berries definitely looks the prettiest, but you can also just stick with one kind of berry. Keep tart covered with plastic wrap in the refrigerator.

Serving Suggestions

The most complementary way to serve this dessert is on a pool of berry sauce accompanied by a dollop of light whipped topping. Crème Anglaise (page 197) is also a nice choice.

Each serving provides

254 Calories   32% Calories from Fat   9 g Fat
38 g Carbohydrates   7 g Protein   91 mg Calcium
3 g Dietary Fiber   267 mg Sodium   31 mg Cholesterol

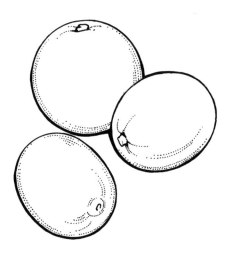

Sweet Deceptions

Lemon Meringue Cheesecake

12 servings

I modeled this cheesecake after the ever-popular lemon meringue pie. There are plenty of lemon cheesecakes out there, but the addition of the meringue makes an unusual and delicious taste and texture.

For crust:

3 whole graham crackers, finely crushed

1/2 cup plain dry bread crumbs

1 1/2 tablespoons light butter, melted

For filling:

2 cups (16 ounces) light Neufchâtel cheese at room temperature

1 1/2 cup (12 ounces) fat-free cream cheese, at room temperature

3/4 cup granulated sugar

1 large whole egg, at room temperature

2 large egg whites, at room temperature

2 tablespoons grated lemon peel

3 tablespoons fresh lemon juice

1 teaspoon lemon extract

2 teaspoons vanilla extract

2 large egg whites, at room temperature

1 tablespoon granulated sugar

For meringue topping:

2 large egg whites, at room temperature

1/4 teaspoon cream of tartar

1/2 cup granulated sugar

continued

Cakes, Tortes, and Tarts

Preheat oven to 350 degrees F. Lightly coat the bottom of an 8-inch or 9-inch springform pan with vegetable or canola oil spray. In a medium-size bowl, combine all the crust ingredients, using your hands to coat the crumbs with butter, making a uniform mixture. Press evenly and firmly into the bottom of prepared pan. Bake for 10 to 15 minutes, until crust is light golden brown and crisp. Set aside to cool while you prepare the filling.

Turn oven down to 325 degrees F. In a large bowl, beat Neufchâtel cheese, cream cheese, and sugar on medium speed of electric mixer until smooth and creamy. Add whole egg, egg whites, lemon peel, lemon juice, lemon extract, and vanilla. Mix just until ingredients are incorporated and batter is smooth.

In a separate, medium-size mixing bowl that is clean and grease-free, beat the remaining 2 egg whites on medium speed of electric mixer until soft peaks form. Increase speed to high and sprinkle in the remaining tablespoon of sugar, beating until firm peaks form. Carefully fold the beaten egg whites into the batter using a rubber spatula. Batter should be uniform, with no streaks of egg white showing. Pour into prepared pan and smooth the top.

Bake for 50 minutes to 1 hour. Cake will be springy when lightly touched in the center, and slightly cracked around the edges due to its lightness. Turn off the oven and allow cake to cool for 1 hour with the oven door ajar. Finish cooling on a rack at room temperature before topping with meringue.

Preheat oven to 375 degrees F. To make the meringue, in a medium-size mixing bowl that is clean and grease-free, beat egg whites with the cream of tartar on medium speed of electric mixer until soft peaks form. Increase speed to high and sprinkle in the sugar a tablespoon at a time, beating until all of the sugar has been incorporated and meringue is stiff and glossy.

Spread meringue over the surface of cheesecake using an icing spatula. If you want any fancy designs on the top, now is the time to do it. Create swirls or peaks using the spatula.

Bake for approximately 10 minutes, or until meringue is light golden brown and crisp. Cool on a rack for 1 hour, then refrigerate for at least 6 hours or overnight before removing from pan and cutting into 12 pieces using the hot-knife method described in General Baking Tips.

Serving Suggestions

This cheesecake is so light and lemony that you may not want to add anything to it at all other than a sprig of mint. I have found it to taste like a whole new dessert when served on a pool of raspberry, strawberry, or orange sauce with some fresh berries.

Each serving provides

258 Calories   37% Calories from Fat   10 g Fat
30 g Carbohydrates   11 g Protein   139 mg Calcium
0 g Dietary Fiber   435 mg Sodium   54 mg Cholesterol

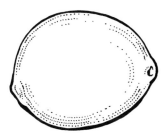

Lemon Raspberry Tart

10 servings

This tart is juicy and refreshing with its combination of tart lemon curd and sweet fresh raspberries. It is the perfect summer dessert, when raspberries are at their best as they are in season.

For crust:

1½ cups all-purpose flour

½ cup powdered sugar, sifted

¼ teaspoon salt

¼ teaspoon baking powder

½ cup (1 stick) light butter, at room temperature

¼ cup (2 ounces) light Neufchâtel cheese, at room temperature

For filling:

2 large whole eggs plus 2 large egg whites, at room temperature

1½ cups granulated sugar

1½ tablespoons grated lemon peel

¼ cup plus 2 tablespoons fresh lemon juice

2½ teaspoons cornstarch

1 pint fresh raspberries

Preheat oven to 350 degrees F. You will need one 9-inch tart pan with removable bottom. In a medium-size bowl combine all the crust ingredients to make a soft pliable dough using one of three methods. I have found the easiest way is in a food processor, fitted with the plastic dough blade, combining all of the ingredients and processing until they form a ball. You can also use a stand mixer with a paddle attachment, mixing all of the ingredients until they form a soft dough. As a last resort, you can combine them by hand.

Place dough on a floured surface and roll out to approximately ⅛-inch thick. Set the tart pan in the center of the rolled-out dough and trim around it with a sharp knife, leaving a 1½-inch border of dough. You will have excess dough that you can roll out to make a few cookies or just wrap and freeze it for another use.

Slide your hands under the circle of dough and place it in the tart pan. This dough is pliable and easy to work with, without the tendency to crack as pie crust does. Press the dough evenly and firmly into all edges of the tart pan. Use a sharp knife to trim off the excess dough flush with the top edge of the pan. Prick crust a few times with a toothpick or skewer and bake for 10 to 15 minutes. Cool on a rack while you prepare the filling.

Preheat oven to 350 degrees F. In a medium-size bowl combine whole eggs, egg whites, and sugar. Whisk together until smooth. Whisk in lemon peel, all the lemon juice, and cornstarch until mixture is smooth and cornstarch has dissolved. Pour into cooled tart shell, still in its pan, and bake for 25 to 30 minutes, until filling is set and no longer liquid. Cool on a rack, and refrigerate for at least 1 hour before finishing tart.

When tart is cold, remove from pan and simply line it with the fresh raspberries all around the outside edge. You should have two rows of berries. Cut tart into 10 slices, using the hot-knife method described in General Baking Tips. Store in an airtight container in the refrigerator.

Each serving provides

239 Calories   20% Calories from Fat   5 g Fat
46 g Carbohydrates   4 g Protein   18 mg Calcium
1 g Dietary Fiber   119 mg Sodium   56 mg Cholesterol

Malted Sponge Cake

12 servings

The texture of this cake is very close to that of angel food cake, only moister and involving fewer headaches as far as procedure is concerned. The malt imparts a mild but distinctive flavor to the finished cake.

Ingredients

1 cup plus 2 tablespoons all-purpose flour
1 teaspoon baking powder
1/2 teaspoon salt
3 large egg yolks, at room temperature
1/2 cup lowfat buttermilk
1 tablespoon vanilla extract

1/4 cup powdered malt (or 2 tablespoons liquid barley malt)
5 large egg whites, at room temperature
1 teaspoon cream of tartar
1 1/4 cups granulated sugar
2 tablespoons powdered sugar, to dust cake

Preheat oven to 350 degrees F. You will need one 10-inch springform pan, ungreased (this allows the batter, which is very light, to climb up the sides of the pan for its height). In a small bowl sift together all the flour, baking powder, and salt. In a large bowl combine egg yolks, buttermilk, vanilla, and malt. Whisk together until smooth. Add sifted dry ingredients and beat on low speed of electric mixer until smooth. Batter may be somewhat thick when using the powdered malt.

In another large mixing bowl that is clean and grease-free, beat the egg whites with the cream of tartar on medium speed of electric mixer until soft peaks form. Increase speed to high and sprinkle in the sugar one tablespoon at a time, beating until all of the sugar has been incorporated and mixture is stiff and glossy. Stir one-fourth of the meringue mixture into the batter, using a rubber spatula to loosen it up. Carefully fold in the remaining meringue. Batter will be very light, and there should be no streaks of egg white showing. However, be very careful not to overfold the batter as this cake depends on the volume from the beaten egg whites. Pour batter into prepared pan and carefully smooth the top with a rubber spatula or an icing spatula.

Bake for 30 to 40 minutes, undisturbed for the first 25 minutes. Cake will be springy when touched lightly in the center, and light golden brown on top. Cool cake in pan upside down on a rack; this method helps to preserve the cake's delicate structure as it cools. I have found that sometimes it will eventually just fall right out of the pan onto the rack, and sometimes it won't. If it does fall out, be sure to invert it upright before cutting. Just slide a sharp knife around the edges before unmolding it. You will see a coating of crumbs left on the entire surface of the pan, which is normal. Cool cake completely before dusting with the powdered sugar, using a fine-mesh sieve. Cut into 12 pieces using a sharp serrated knife. Store in an airtight container.

Serving Suggestions

The possibilities for this cake are endless. I left the recipe very simple because after tasting it for the first time, my husband and I devoured half the cake inside of two hours. We decided it was good enough to stand on its own, with the option of elaborating on it. So far I have filled it with such things as fresh berries and light whipped topping. I have also sliced it into three even layers with a sharp serrated knife and filled them with chocolate ganache and/or raspberry jam. Try serving it on berry sauces, or even the Gooey Caramel Sauce (page 198). If you would like to change the flavor and texture of the cake a little, add 1/2 cup ground toasted nuts of your choice to the sifted dry ingredients before incorporating them into the liquid mixture.

Each serving provides

163 Calories   8% Calories from Fat   2 g Fat
34 g Carbohydrates   4 g Protein   25 mg Calcium
0 g Dietary Fiber   206 mg Sodium   54 mg Cholesterol

Pear Pound Cake

12 servings

This cake is made with dried pears, not fresh, simply because of their intensity. Opt for unsulphured pears, if you can find them. The resulting very moist cake demands a dollop of light whipped topping, along with a generous drizzling of Gem Caramel (page 200) for a truly decadent treat.

Ingredients

6 dried pear halves (8 if pears are small in size)

1 cup water

2 tablespoons granulated sugar

2 cups all-purpose flour

1 teaspoon salt

2 teaspoons baking powder

1 teaspoon ground ginger

1/2 teaspoon ground allspice

1/2 cup lowfat ricotta cheese

3/4 cup plus 2 tablespoons granulated sugar

1/4 cup (1/2 stick) light butter, at room temperature

1/4 cup honey

2 large egg whites, at room temperature

2 teaspoons vanilla extract

1/4 cup milk (2 percent)

Preheat oven to 350 degrees F. Lightly coat a 9 × 2-inch or 10 x 2-inch springform pan with vegetable or canola oil spray and dust with flour.

Chop the dried pears into 1/2-inch pieces, removing any hard parts of the core. In a small saucepan combine the pears with the water and 2 tablespoons sugar. Simmer over medium heat for 12 to 15 minutes to soften them. Remove from heat and set aside to cool.

Place cooled pears and any remaining liquid in a food processor fitted with the metal blade and puree until smooth. Measure out enough pear puree to make one cup. If it comes out a little bit short, just add some extra lowfat ricotta to bring it up to one cup.

In a small bowl, combine flour, salt, baking powder, ginger, and allspice. In a large mixing bowl, cream ricotta, the remaining sugar, and butter on medium speed of electric mixer until smooth. Beat in the honey, egg whites, vanilla and pear puree until smooth and incorporated. On low speed, add the dry ingredients alternately with the milk, beating until batter is smooth. Batter will be somewhat thick. Pour into prepared pan and smooth the top with a rubber spatula.

Bake for 40 to 45 minutes, or until a cake tester comes out clean or with just a few moist crumbs on it. Cool completely in pan on a rack before removing from pan and cutting into 12 slices. Store in an airtight container in the refrigerator, and serve at room temperature.

Serving Suggestions

This cake loves to be served with light whipped topping and Gem Caramel Sauce (page 200). You can also serve it on Crème Anglaise (page 197) and sprinkle it with cinnamon.

Each serving provides

198 Calories   13% Calories from Fat   3 g Fat
41 g Carbohydrates   4 g Protein   62 mg Calcium
1 g Dietary Fiber   261 mg Sodium   10 mg Cholesterol

Strawberry Amaretto Shortcakes

10 servings

These tender buttermilk scones are filled with amaretto-marinated strawberries and light whipped topping. These treats have a nice old-fashioned appeal and a comforting flavor.

For buttermilk scones:

2 cups all-purpose flour	3/4 cup lowfat buttermilk
1/2 teaspoon salt	1/4 cup lowfat ricotta cheese
1 tablespoon baking powder	2 teaspoons vanilla extract
2 tablespoons granulated sugar	1 egg white, beaten until frothy
1/4 cup butter-flavored vegetable shortening	2 tablespoons granulated sugar for topping scones

For amaretto strawberries:

2 pounds fresh strawberries, hulled and sliced 1/4 inch thick	1/4 cup almond liqueur (Amaretto)
1/3 cup granulated sugar	1 teaspoon vanilla extract

For assembly:

2 1/2 cups light whipped topping

Preheat oven to 400 degrees F. Line a cookie sheet with foil or parchment paper. To make shortcakes, in a large bowl combine flour, salt, baking powder, and 2 tablespoons sugar. Add the shortening and rub the mixture together with your fingers to completely distribute shortening; mixture will be coarse.

In a medium-size bowl, whisk together buttermilk, ricotta, and vanilla until smooth. Pour into dry ingredients and mix with a fork to form a soft dough. Turn dough out onto a floured board and knead slightly to form a ball. Roll or pat dough out to a 9-inch circle. Brush top of dough with the beaten egg white and sprinkle with the remaining 2 tablespoons sugar. Cut dough into 10 even wedges, using a sharp knife. Place wedges at least 1 inch apart on prepared cookie sheet and bake for 20 to 25 minutes, or until scones are light golden brown. Cool completely on a rack.

To prepare the strawberries, in a large bowl combine strawberries, sugar, Amaretto, and vanilla. Cover and refrigerate for 1 hour to develop flavors.

For final assembly, slice each scone in half horizontally with a serrated knife. Fill each scone with approximately half a cup of the berries and spoon about a quarter cup of the whipped topping over each lid. If making these ahead of time, store scones in an airtight container at room temperature and the berries in an airtight container in the refrigerator.

Serving Suggestions

For the ultimate finishing touch, serve these on a pool of fresh Strawberry Sauce (page 203), and maybe a few chocolate curls on top of the whipped topping. For a different approach, try the Orange Sauce (page 204), as strawberries and oranges go very well together.

Each serving provides

286 Calories   33% Calories from Fat   10 g Fat
45 g Carbohydrates   5 g Protein   93 mg Calcium
3 g Dietary Fiber   245 mg Sodium   3 mg Cholesterol

Toasted Hazelnut Marble Cheesecake

16 servings

The toasted hazelnuts give this cheesecake an elegant taste, and it goes perfectly with a cup of dark espresso.

For crust:

3 whole graham crackers, finely crushed

1/2 cup plain dry bread crumbs

1/4 teaspoon ground cinnamon

1 1/2 tablespoons light butter, melted

For hazelnut marble:

2 ounces (approximately 1/2 cup) ground toasted hazelnuts

2 tablespoons firmly packed brown sugar

1 teaspoon all-purpose flour

1/8 teaspoon salt

1 large egg white, at room temperature

1 tablespoon dark corn syrup

1/4 teaspoon vanilla extract

For filling:

2 cups (16 ounces) light Neufchâtel cheese, at room temperature

1 1/2 cups (12 ounces) fat-free cream cheese, at room temperature

3/4 cup granulated sugar

2 large whole eggs, at room temperature

1 tablespoon vanilla extract

2 tablespoons hazelnut liqueur such as frangelico

3 large egg whites, at room temperature

1 tablespoon granulated sugar

Preheat oven to 350 degrees F. Lightly coat the bottom of an 8-inch or 9-inch springform pan with vegetable or canola oil spray. In a small bowl combine all the crust ingredients, using your hands to coat the crumbs with the butter to make a uniform mixture. Press evenly and firmly into the bottom of prepared pan. Bake for 10 to 15 minutes, until crust is light golden brown and crisp. Set aside to cool while you prepare the marble.

In a small bowl combine hazelnuts, brown sugar, flour, and salt. Stir in egg white, corn syrup, and vanilla until smooth. Set aside to prepare filling.

Preheat oven to 325 degrees F. In a large mixing bowl cream Neufchâtel cheese, cream cheese, and the sugar on medium speed of electric mixer until smooth. Add whole eggs, vanilla, and hazelnut liqueur, mixing just until eggs are incorporated and batter is smooth.

In a separate medium-size mixing bowl that is clean and grease-free, beat the egg whites on medium speed of electric mixer until soft peaks form. Increase speed to high and sprinkle in remaining tablespoon of sugar, beating until firm peaks form. Carefully fold the beaten egg whites into the batter with a rubber spatula. Batter should be uniform, with no streaks of egg white showing.

Pour batter into prepared pan and smooth the top. Dot the surface with the hazelnut mixture and use an icing spatula or a knife to swirl it into the batter for a marbled look.

Bake for 50 minutes to 1 hour. Cake will be springy when lightly touched in the center, and slightly cracked around the edges due to its lightness. Turn off the oven and allow cake to cool for 1 hour with the oven door ajar. Finish cooling on a rack at room temperature, then refrigerate for at least 6 hours or overnight

continued

Cakes, Tortes, and Tarts

before removing from pan and cutting into 16 slices using the hot-knife method described in General Baking Tips. Store in an airtight container in the refrigerator.

Serving Suggestions

This cheesecake can be deliciously accented in a number of ways. Try pairing it up with Chocolate or Caramel Sauce (pages 201, 200). For a sophisticated taste, try Coffee Anglaise (a variation on page 197) under it. Extra toasted nuts are always a plus.

Each serving provides

216 Calories   44% Calories from Fat   11 g Fat
20 g Carbohydrates   9 g Protein   114 mg Calcium
0 g Dietary Fiber   332 mg Sodium   55 mg Cholesterol

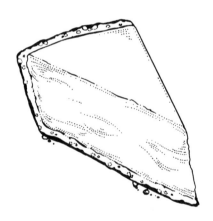

Tunnel of Peanut Butter Cake

16 servings

When I was a kid, we used to eat a cake called Tunnel of Fudge. It was a moist devil's food cake with a tunnel of rich, creamy fudge running right through the middle. It was baked in a bundt pan so the filling was visible in each slice. This memory was my inspiration for the Tunnel of Peanut Butter, a moist chocolate cake with a tunnel of creamy peanut butter filling, and chocolate icing running down its sides!

For peanut butter tunnel:

- 1/4 cup firmly packed brown sugar
- 1 tablespoon granulated sugar
- 1 tablespoon all-purpose flour
- 1/4 cup plus 1 tablespoon reduced-fat peanut butter
- 1/2 cup plus 2 tablespoons (5 ounces) fat-free cream cheese, at room temperature
- 1/2 teaspoon vanilla extract

For chocolate cake:

- 2 1/2 cups all-purpose flour
- 1/2 cup unsweetened cocoa
- 1 tablespoon baking powder
- 1/2 teaspoon salt
- 1 1/2 cups granulated sugar
- 1/2 cup (1 stick) light butter, at room temperature
- 2 tablespoons lowfat ricotta cheese
- 2 large egg whites, at room temperature
- 1 tablespoon vanilla extract
- 1 tablespoon cider vinegar
- 1/2 cup lowfat buttermilk
- 1/3 cup milk (2 percent)

continued

For chocolate icing:

1 cup powdered sugar, sifted

2 tablespoons unsweetened cocoa, sifted

2½ tablespoons milk (2 percent)

In a small mixing bowl combine all the tunnel ingredients and beat on medium speed of electric mixer until smooth and creamy. Set aside while you make the cake.

Preheat oven to 350 degrees F. Lightly coat a large bundt pan with vegetable or canola oil spray and dust with flour. In a small bowl combine flour, cocoa, baking powder, and salt. Set aside.

In a large mixing bowl cream sugar, butter, and ricotta on medium speed of electric mixer until smooth. Beat in egg whites, vanilla, and vinegar. Beat in buttermilk. Add dry ingredients alternately with the 2 percent milk, and beat on medium speed until batter is smooth.

Pour half of the batter into prepared pan and tap pan lightly on counter to level it out. Spoon the peanut butter mixture as evenly as you can onto the center of the filling, all the way around the pan. It will rest right on top of the batter. You can also put filling in a pastry bag without the tip and pipe it onto the batter. Pour the remaining cake batter over top of the peanut butter tunnel, using a spatula to disperse it evenly and enclose the peanut butter filling.

Bake for 35 to 40 minutes. Cake will spring back when lightly touched in center. Turn cake out onto a rack and cool completely before icing.

To make the icing, combine all the icing ingredients in a small bowl and stir until creamy. Use a spoon to drizzle icing over cake. If it is too thick, add another teaspoon of milk until consistency is right. Store cake in an airtight container in the refrigerator. Cake tastes best when brought to room temperature before serving.

Be sure to sprinkle some chopped peanuts over the icing before it sets. You could also serve this cake on a pool of Chocolate or Caramel Sauce (page 201, 200).

Each serving provides

270 Calories   20% Calories from Fat   6 g Fat
49 g Carbohydrates   7 g Protein   80 mg Calcium
1 g Dietary Fiber   270 mg Sodium   13 mg Cholesterol

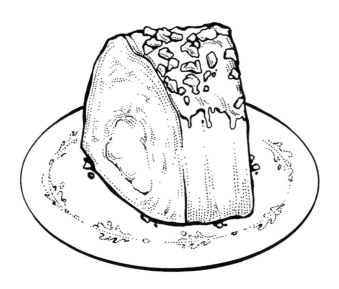

Cakes, Tortes, and Tarts

White Chocolate Raspberry Revel

16 servings

As far as I'm concerned, there just aren't enough white chocolate desserts out there. I think they often get passed by for the dark versions. White chocolate has a decadence all its own, as you will soon experience with this moist white chocolate cake, layered with heavenly raspberry buttercream, fresh raspberries, and luscious white chocolate curls!

For cake:

- 3/4 cup milk (2 percent)
- 4 ounces white chocolate, chopped
- 1 1/2 cups all-purpose flour
- 2 teaspoons baking powder
- 1/2 teaspoon salt
- 1/4 cup (1 ounce) finely ground blanched almonds
- 1 cup granulated sugar
- 2 tablespoons vegetable shortening

- 1/2 cup lowfat ricotta cheese
- 1 tablespoon vanilla extract
- 2 large egg whites, at room temperature

- 3 large egg whites, at room temperature
- 1/8 teaspoon cream of tartar
- 1/4 cup granulated sugar

For raspberry buttercream:

- 1/2 cup granulated sugar
- 1/4 cup water
- 1/4 cup seedless raspberry jam
- 1/3 cup (approximately 3 large) egg whites, at room temperature
- 1/8 teaspoon cream of tartar

- 1 tablespoon granulated sugar
- 1/2 cup (1 stick) unsalted, butter at room temperature
- 3 tablespoons vegetable shortening, at room temperature

For assembly:

1/4 cup seedless raspberry
     jam
1 cup fresh raspberries

powdered sugar to
dust top
white chocolate curls,
optional (page 191)

Preheat oven to 350 degrees F. Lightly coat two 8 × 2-inch baking pans with vegetable or canola oil spray and dust with flour.

To prepare cake, in a small saucepan combine milk and white chocolate. Use a wire whisk, it helps distribute the chocolate. Cook over low heat, stirring occasionally, until chocolate has completely melted into the milk. Remove from heat and cool to room temperature.

In a small bowl combine flour, baking powder, salt, and ground almonds. In a large bowl cream the 1 cup sugar, shortening, and ricotta on medium speed of electric mixer until smooth. Add vanilla and the 2 egg whites and beat until fully incorporated. Whisk in the white chocolate mixture; it will appear curdled but will smooth out with addition of the flour. On low speed gradually beat in the dry ingredients until batter is smooth.

In a medium-size mixing bowl that is clean and grease-free, beat the remaining 3 egg whites with the cream of tartar on medium speed of electric mixer until soft peaks form. Increase speed to high and sprinkle in the 1/4 cup of sugar a tablespoon at a time, beating until all of the sugar has been incorporated and firm peaks have formed. The egg whites will look slightly glossy. Carefully fold beaten egg whites into the batter using a rubber spatula.

Divide batter evenly between the two prepared pans and bake for 25 to 30 minutes, or until a cake tester inserted into the center

continued

Cakes, Tortes, and Tarts

comes out clean. Immediately turn cakes out onto racks to cool. Cool cakes completely before assembling and frosting.

To make the buttercream, in a small saucepan combine the 1/2 cup sugar, water, and raspberry jam, and place over high heat. As mixture begins to warm up, use a whisk to dissolve the jam into the sugar. Clip a candy thermometer onto the pan and cook mixture undisturbed until the candy thermometer reads 235 degrees F. This is just before the soft ball stage. It is important to take the sugar off the heat before it gets to the soft ball stage of 240 degrees F, because at that critical point the jam begins to caramelize and subsequently burn. Timing is everything here, but not difficult. The sugar takes approximately 5 to 7 minutes to reach the proper temperature. Once you have it over the heat and it is bubbling, watch the thermometer.

Meanwhile, combine the egg whites and cream of tartar in a medium-size bowl that is clean and grease-free. When the sugar syrup reaches about 200 degrees F, start beating the egg whites on medium speed of electric mixer until soft peaks form. Increase speed to high and sprinkle in the remaining tablespoon of sugar, beating until firm peaks form.

By now the syrup should be at the proper temperature to be incorporated. Pour the hot syrup into the egg whites in a slow, steady stream while beating on high speed. The syrup will be somewhat thick, but it ends up working its way into the egg whites without a problem. Continue to beat, moving the beaters around to evenly distribute the syrup if using a hand mixer. Beat mixture until it is room temperature to the touch, and stiff and glossy.

At this point, slow the mixer down to medium speed and add the butter and shortening all at once. Once they have been incorporated, increase the speed to high again and continue to beat until icing is fluffy. It is important that the egg whites not be warm when you add the butter, or the icing will become curdled and soupy, due to the melting of the butter. If this does happen, you can still save the batch of icing as long as it is only slightly soupy, and not a full-blown, curdled mess! Simply beat in more butter or shortening, a little at a time, until the icing comes together and firms up. This may change your calorie and fat counts a bit, but it's better than starting all over again.

When it's finally assembled, this torte is intended to look rustic and imperfect. No pastry bags with fancy tips allowed! The icing should ooze out the sides, and the top should be mounded with fresh raspberries and white chocolate curls.

Use a serrated knife to trim off the tops of the cooled cakes, exposing their inner structure so they can absorb the jam filling. Place one cake layer exposed side up on a cardboard circle or plate. Spread it with the 1/4 cup jam, using a metal icing spatula. Go over the jam a few times with the spatula to mash it into all those little holes in the cake.

Carefully spread half of the raspberry buttercream over the jam layer, all the way to the edges. Top with the second cake layer, exposed side down. Press down on the cake gently, just enough to make the icing reach the edges. Spread the remaining buttercream over the top of the cake. As another option, you may spread raspberry jam on the top layer as well before adding buttercream.

Top with the fresh raspberries and dust with powdered sugar. For the full effect, throw on some of those optional white chocolate curls (page 191) and then dust with powdered sugar. This cake should be served at room temperature in order to fully appreciate its flavor and texture. However, it should be stored in the refrigerator in an airtight container because the raspberries are perishable.

Serving Suggestions

The only other thing I would do with this cake is serve it on a pool of Raspberry Sauce (page 202).

Each serving provides

318 Calories   40% Calories from Fat   14 g Fat
45 g Carbohydrates   5 g Protein   75 mg Calcium
1 g Dietary Fiber   158 mg Sodium   21 mg Cholesterol

Cookies, Bars, and Squares

Chocolate Chip Cookies

Coconut Raspberry Macaroons

Chocolate Crinkles

Oatmeal and Chocolate Chip Cookies

PB & J Kisses

Pistachio Chocolate Cookies

Sugared Hazelnut Biscuits

Cakey Brownies

Cakey Brownies with Creamy Peanut Butter Icing

Chocolate Peanut Butter Brownies

Fudgy Brownies

Turtle Brownies

Apple Raisin Oatmeal Bars

Carrot Cake Squares with Cream Cheese Frosting

Caramel Coconut Bars

Key Lime Squares

Luscious Lemon Squares

Peanut Butter Cookies

Chapter Four

Cookies, Bars, and Squares

At times everyone's sweet tooth needs just a little nibble to keep it happy. I find cookies, brownies, and dessert-type bars to be the perfect fix, especially for that mid-afternoon sugar craving so many of us seem to get whether we are at work or play! So I have included some of my personal favorites in this book because life just wouldn't be complete without them. Though these nibbles are of the lowfat variety, they are just as easy to bake successfully as regular cookies and bars. The following tips will be helpful when making these recipes.

Pan Preparation

Most of the cookie recipes will ask you to line the cookie sheet with foil or parchment paper and lightly coat with nonstick cooking spray. You'll find a description of parchment paper in the beginning of the book in Equipment descriptions. Most people have aluminum foil around and I find it to be more than satisfactory for lining my cookie sheets. Lightly coating the foil or parchment paper with the nonstick cooking spray is my way of guaranteeing that those cookies will come right off the cookie sheet without any hassles, especially since these cookies are not made with large amounts of butter or shortening to aid in their release from the pan. For the brownies and other squares and bars, the pans are all coated with nonstick vegetable or canola oil spray, and only a couple of them require a light dusting of flour.

Mixing Cookie Doughs

In General Baking Tips, I mentioned that I relied on a good-quality hand mixer for my mixing needs in this book except for the stiffer cookie doughs. I would like to elaborate a bit on that particular subject. If you happen to own a stand mixer that is meant for heavy-duty jobs like mixing cookie doughs, then go ahead and use it, but the recipes in this book will come out just as well if you have to use a wooden spoon and a little elbow grease when it comes to stirring in flour, which is exactly what I did for the cookies in this book. All you really have to do is make sure all the ingredients are well combined, no matter how you choose to combine them.

Measuring the Dough

Why does a recipe show a yield of 3 dozen cookies and you only get 2 1/2 dozen? I couldn't leave this subject alone, because this is a common occurrence, but I assure you it shouldn't be a problem in this book. I could ask ten people to drop the dough by the tablespoonful, and I don't think anyone would come out with the same number of cookies. Everyone has their own interpretation of what a tablespoon is so as long as you're close that's fine! One or two cookies more or less isn't going change the numbers that drastically so don't worry if you don't come out with the exact number of cookies that I do.

Baking Times and Temperatures

All of the cookies and bars are baked at the standard 350 degrees Fahrenheit. For the cookies, you'll find that each recipe asks you to bake them for an approximate time or until they are light golden brown. Don't let them cook to a really dark brown or they will be overcooked. I suggest looking at them and lightly touching them when they are within a few minutes of the suggested time. You can probably make a pretty close assessment how much longer they need to bake, when they're no longer gooey in the middle.

Brownie Tips

Coming up with a lowfat brownie recipe that could effectively substitute for the real thing was no easy task, and I want to pass along to you some information that will help ensure your brownies will come out the way they are supposed to. Because these brownies are missing all that butter found in most brownies, it is quite a bit easier to overbake them. Perfect timing is critical for making a lowfat brownie that is just as moist as its fattening counterpart. I have found it best to slightly underbake my brownies to get the moist texture we all love. Easier said than done, especially if you have a temperamental oven! If a recipe says to bake for approximately 17 to 20 minutes, I would check them at the 17-minute mark because they may very well be done. Avoid the temptation to bake them until they are firm to the touch; they should still be slightly soft when you press lightly in the middle. You will develop a feel for it after making them a couple of times. I like my brownies gooey and I will purposely underbake them by as much as 5 minutes, depending on the recipe, but if you like them to be cakier in texture, go ahead and bake them for the allotted time.

Airtight Containers

There is no doubt that Tupperware-type containers are best, especially when it comes to brownies and bars. But the trusty old Ziploc bag is my second choice for keeping these treats fresh. Some of the cookies and bars that have soft toppings or delicate dustings of sugar should be kept in a Tupperware-type container so they don't get squashed. You can also keep them wrapped in plastic on a plate.

Chocolate Chip Cookies

32 cookies

Where would we be without this all-American classic? I shudder to think! This version is lighter in texture than most chocolate chip cookies, but you won't be missing out on any of the flavor.

Ingredients

2 1/4 cups all-purpose flour
1 teaspoon baking soda
3/4 teaspoon salt
5 tablespoons mini semi-sweet chocolate chips
3/4 cup firmly packed brown sugar
1/2 cup granulated sugar
1/2 cup (1 stick) light butter at room temperature
1 tablespoon dark corn syrup
1/2 cup fat-free ricotta cheese
1 tablespoon vanilla extract
1 large egg white, at room temperature

Preheat oven to 350 degrees F. Line a cookie sheet with foil or parchment paper and lightly coat with nonstick vegetable or canola oil spray. In a small bowl combine flour, baking soda, salt, and chocolate chips.

In a large bowl cream sugars, butter, corn syrup, and ricotta on medium speed of electric mixer until smooth. Beat in vanilla and egg white. Stir in dry ingredients until thoroughly combined.

Drop dough by the tablespoonful 1 1/2 inches apart onto prepared cookie sheet. Bake 8 to 10 minutes, until light golden brown. Cool completely on a rack and store in an airtight container.

Each serving provides

92 Calories   22% Calories from Fat   2 g Fat
17 g Carbohydrates   2 g Protein   20 mg Calcium
0 g Dietary Fiber   116 mg Sodium   6 mg Cholesterol

Coconut Raspberry Macaroons

36 cookies

Here is a nice change from plain coconut macaroons. The raspberry jam gives them a mild, fruity taste. They are even better when dipped in dark chocolate.

Ingredients

5 large egg whites, at room temperature	2 teaspoons vanilla extract
1½ cups powdered sugar	1 cup all-purpose flour
3 tablespoons seedless red raspberry jam	1 (14-ounce) bag sweetened flaked coconut

Preheat oven to 350 degrees F. Line a cookie sheet with foil or parchment paper and lightly coat with vegetable or canola oil spray.

In a large bowl combine egg whites and sugar. Whisk together until smooth and creamy. Whisk in raspberry jam and vanilla. Don't worry if jam does not completely blend into the egg white mixture. Stir in flour until smooth and then stir in the coconut until fully incorporated.

Drop dough by the tablespoonful 1½ inches apart onto prepared cookie sheet. Bake for 15 to 20 minutes or until light golden brown. Cool completely on a rack and store in an airtight container.

Each serving provides

93 Calories   39% Calories from Fat   4 g Fat
14 g Carbohydrates   1 g Protein   3 mg Calcium
1 g Dietary Fiber   37 mg Sodium   0 mg Cholesterol

Chocolate Crinkles

32 cookies

These cookies are my favorite! My mother-in-law serves them every Christmas and I can easily make a plate of them disappear all on my own. They are moist and cakey, with just the right amount of chocolate. Great with a cup of coffee!

Ingredients

3/4 cup all-purpose flour

1/3 cup whole wheat flour

1/3 cup unsweetened cocoa, sifted

1/2 teaspoon baking powder

1/4 teaspoon baking soda

2 1/2 tablespoons finely ground almonds

1/4 cup (1/2 stick) light butter, at room temperature

3/4 cup granulated sugar

1/2 cup plus 2 tablespoons small-curd, lowfat cottage cheese

2 large egg whites, at room temperature

2 1/2 teaspoons vanilla extract

1 3/4 cups sifted powdered sugar

Preheat oven to 350 degrees F. Line a cookie sheet with foil or parchment paper and lightly coat with vegetable or canola oil spray. In a small bowl combine both flours, cocoa, baking powder, baking soda, and ground almonds.

In a medium-size bowl combine the butter, sugar, and cottage cheese. Beat on medium speed of electric mixer for approximately 30 seconds. It's okay if some of the cheese curds are still whole; they will eventually get worked into the dough. Add the egg whites and vanilla and beat just enough to incorporate them. Stir in the flour mixture to make a soft, sticky dough and refrigerate for 3 hours or overnight. Chilling the dough makes it much easier to work with.

Place powdered sugar in a shallow bowl or spread it out on a plate. Using a small spoon, scoop up 1-inch balls of the chilled dough and drop them in the sugar. Roll each one between the

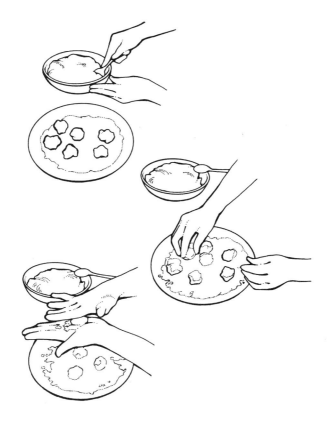

palms of your hands to make a ball. Roll the balls in the sugar once more before placing them 1 1/2 inches apart on prepared cookie sheet.

Bake for 10 to 12 minutes. They will look crinkled and be firm to the touch. Cool completely on a rack and store in an airtight container, separating the layers with waxed paper if you are stacking them.

Each serving provides

71 Calories   19% Calories from Fat   2 g Fat
14 g Carbohydrates   2 g Protein   8 mg Calcium
0 g Dietary Fiber   49 mg Sodium   3 mg Cholesterol

Cookies, Bars, and Squares

Oatmeal and Chocolate Chip Cookies

40 cookies

These treats are moist and chewy, as oatmeal cookies should be. They always find their way into our backpacks when we go hiking.

Ingredients

2 cups all-purpose flour	1/2 cup granulated sugar
1/2 teaspoon salt	1/2 cup (1 stick) light butter, at room temperature
1 teaspoon ground allspice	
1/2 teaspoon ground ginger	1/2 cup honey
1 teaspoon baking soda	1/4 cup fat-free ricotta cheese
2 1/2 cups old-fashioned oats	
5 tablespoons mini semi-sweet chocolate chips	2 large egg whites, at room temperature
1 cup firmly packed brown sugar	2 teaspoons vanilla extract

Preheat oven to 350 degrees F. Line a cookie sheet with foil or parchment paper and lightly coat with nonstick cooking spray. In a medium-size bowl combine flour, salt, spices, baking soda, oats, and chocolate chips.

In a large bowl cream both sugars, butter, honey, and ricotta on medium speed of electric mixer until smooth. Beat in egg whites and vanilla until fully incorporated. Stir in dry ingredients and drop dough by the tablespoonful 2 inches apart onto prepared cookie sheet.

Bake for 10 to 12 minutes, until cookies are light golden brown. Cool completely on a rack and store in an airtight container.

Variation

Oatmeal Raisin Cookies: Substitute 3/4 cup chopped raisins or sultanas for the chocolate chips.

Each serving provides

106 Calories   17% Calories from Fat   2 g Fat
21 g Carbohydrates   2 g Protein   16 mg Calcium
1 g Dietary Fiber   85 mg Sodium   4 mg Cholesterol

(Variation) Each serving provides

118 Calories   12% Calories from Fat   2 g Fat
23 g Carbohydrates   4 g Protein   51 mg Calcium
1 g Dietary Fiber   109 mg Sodium   6 mg Cholesterol

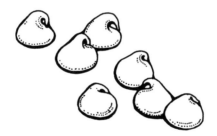

Cookies, Bars, and Squares

PB & J Kisses

60 cookies

These cookies are my husband's favorite and I have gotten into the habit of hiding half of them, otherwise he eats every one! These are chewy peanut butter cookies filled with your favorite jam, reminiscent of mini peanut butter and jelly sandwiches.

Ingredients

1 1/4 cups all-purpose flour

1/2 cup whole wheat flour

1/2 teaspoon baking soda

1/2 cup firmly packed brown sugar

1/2 cup granulated sugar plus 1/3 cup, for rolling cookies

6 tablespoons (3/4 stick) light butter, at room temperature

1 cup reduced-fat peanut butter

2 large egg whites, at room temperature

2 teaspoons vanilla extract

6 tablespoons jam or jelly, any flavor

Preheat oven to 350 degrees F. Line a cookie sheet with foil or parchment paper. In a small bowl combine both flours and baking soda.

In a large mixing bowl cream both sugars, butter, and peanut butter on medium speed of electric mixer until smooth. Beat in egg whites and vanilla until fully incorporated. Stir in dry ingredients to make a soft dough.

Roll dough into 1-inch balls, roll in sugar, and place 2 inches apart on prepared cookie sheet. Indent the center of each cookie with your finger and fill the indentation with approximately 1/4 teaspoon of jam or jelly.

Bake for 10 to 12 minutes or until light golden brown and jam is melted and bubbly around the edges. Cool completely on a rack and store in an airtight container.

Each serving provides

61 Calories   30% Calories from Fat   2 g Fat
10 g Carbohydrates   2 g Protein   3 mg Calcium
0 g Dietary Fiber   42 mg Sodium   2 mg Cholesterol

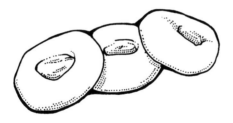

Pistachio Chocolate Cookies

30 cookies

These cookies are very much like the Chocolate Crinkles in taste and texture. The addition of the pistachios produces a sophisticated flavor and appearance with the bright green standing out against the chocolate. These are great after-dinner cookies to serve with coffee when you don't want a whole dessert.

Ingredients

1 1/2 cups all-purpose flour
3/4 teaspoon baking soda
1/4 teaspoon salt
1 cup granulated sugar
1/3 cup light butter, at room temperature
1/2 cup small-curd, lowfat cottage cheese
1 large whole egg, at room temperature

1 tablespoon vanilla extract
2 tablespoons unsweetened cocoa, sifted
3 tablespoons finely ground pistachios
green food color, optional
chopped pistachios for sprinkling tops, optional

Preheat oven to 350 degrees F. Line a cookie sheet with aluminum foil or parchment paper and lightly coat with vegetable or canola oil spray. In a small bowl combine flour, baking soda, and salt.

In a medium-size mixing bowl cream sugar, butter, and cottage cheese on medium speed of electric mixer until smooth. Add the egg and vanilla, and beat until fully incorporated. Stir in the dry ingredients to make a soft dough.

Divide dough in half. Into one half stir the ground pistachios, and to the other half add the cocoa. You now have two different colors of dough. If you would like to accentuate the green of the pistachios, add a drop of green food color when mixing them in; this makes a very colorful cookie.

Drop the chocolate dough by the heaping teaspoonful 2 inches apart onto prepared cookie sheet. Place a heaping teaspoonful of the pistachio dough directly on top of each chocolate drop, flattening it just a bit so it stays on top when baking.

Bake for approximately 12 minutes. Cookies should be firm to the touch. Cool completely on a rack and store in an airtight container. As an added touch, sprinkle the cookies with a few chopped pistachios before baking.

Each serving provides

67 Calories 24% Calories from Fat 2 g Fat
12 g Carbohydrates 2 g Protein 5 mg Calcium
0 g Dietary Fiber 79 mg Sodium 10 mg Cholesterol

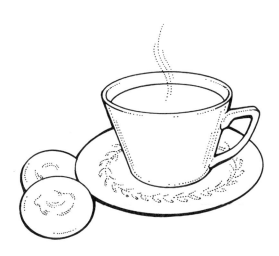

Sugared Hazelnut Biscuits

48 cookies

If you are a fan of biscotti, I urge you to give these biscuits a try. I created these specifically with lattes and espressos in mind. The difference here is that you won't chip a tooth, as these are soft, with a mild hazelnut flavor.

Ingredients

2³/4   cups all-purpose flour
 ¹/2   teaspoon salt
1¹/2   teaspoons baking soda
   2   ounces (¹/2 cup) finely ground toasted hazelnuts
1¹/4   cups granulated sugar plus ¹/4 cup for dusting cookies
 ¹/2   cup (1 stick) light butter, at room temperature

 ¹/2   cup fat-free ricotta cheese
   1   large egg white, at room temperature
   1   tablespoon vanilla extract
1¹/2   teaspoons hazelnut liqueur such as frangelico

Preheat oven to 350 degrees F. Line a cookie sheet with foil or parchment paper and lightly coat with vegetable or canola oil spray. In a small bowl combine flour, salt, baking soda, and hazelnuts.

In a large mixing bowl cream the 1¹/4 cups sugar, butter, and ricotta on medium speed of electric mixer until smooth. Beat in egg white, vanilla, and hazelnut liqueur until fully incorporated. Stir in dry ingredients to make a soft dough.

Divide dough in half and roll each half into a log 9 to 10 inches long. Place each log on a piece of plastic wrap. With floured hands pat it into a nice even rectangle about 4 inches wide. Cover rectangles with plastic wrap, place on a cookie sheet, and freeze for at least 2 hours or overnight.

When ready to bake cookies, slice each rectangle into 24 oblong cookies using a sharp knife. Cookies should be 4 inches long

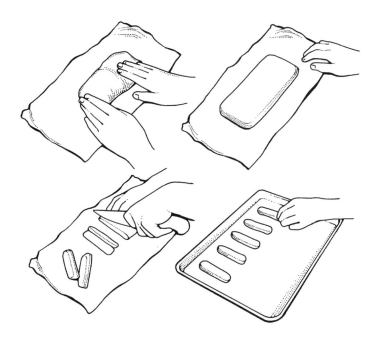

and approximately ¼-inch thick. Coat cookies with remaining sugar before placing 1½ inches apart on prepared cookie sheet. Bake for 15 to 17 minutes, or until light golden brown. Cool completely on a rack and store in an airtight container.

Each serving provides

69 Calories   24% Calories from Fat   2 g Fat
12 g Carbohydrates   1 g Protein   12 mg Calcium
0 g Dietary Fiber   50 mg Sodium   4 mg Cholesterol

Cakey Brownies

16 brownies

Ingredients

3/4 cup all-purpose flour

1/4 teaspoon baking soda

3/4 teaspoon salt

2 ounces (2 squares) unsweetened chocolate

1/2 cup plus 1 tablespoon dark corn syrup

1 tablespoon canola oil

1/4 cup fat-free ricotta cheese

3/4 cup granulated sugar

1 large whole egg plus 1 large egg white, at room temperature

1 tablespoon vanilla extract

Preheat oven to 350 degrees F. Lightly coat an 8 × 8 × 2-inch baking pan with vegetable or canola oil spray. In a small bowl combine flour, baking soda, and salt.

In a small saucepan combine chocolate, corn syrup, and oil. Melt over low heat, stirring until smooth. Remove from heat and cool for 10 minutes.

In a medium-size bowl combine ricotta, sugar, whole egg, egg white, and vanilla, and whisk together until smooth. Whisk in cooled chocolate mixture. Stir in dry ingredients to make a smooth batter. Pour into prepared pan.

Bake for 17 to 20 minutes. Cake should indent slightly when touched in the center. Cool completely in pan, on a rack, before cutting into 16 squares using the hot-knife method described in General Baking Tips. Store in an airtight container.

Each serving provides

125 Calories   22% Calories from Fat   3 g Fat
24 g Carbohydrates   2 g Protein   19 mg Calcium
0 g Dietary Fiber   153 mg Sodium   14 mg Cholesterol

Cakey Brownies with Creamy Peanut Butter Icing

16 brownies

The addition of peanut butter icing to these already moist and chocolatey brownies makes them quite a decadent treat. Peanut butter and chocolate were made for each other. Make sure you have plenty of milk to wash these down!

Ingredients

One recipe of Cakey Brownies, completely cooled and still in the pan
1 cup powdered sugar
1 1/2 tablespoons reduced-fat peanut butter

2 tablespoons light butter, at room temperature
1 tablespoon light corn syrup
1/2 teaspoon vanilla extract
1 1/2 teaspoons water

Combine all the icing ingredients in a small bowl and beat on medium speed of an electric mixer for 2 to 3 minutes until smooth and creamy. Spread evenly over cooled cake and cut into 16 squares using the hot-knife method described in General Baking Tips. Store in an airtight container.

Each serving provides

137 Calories   29% Calories from Fat   4 g Fat
23 g Carbohydrates   3 g Protein   19 mg Calcium
0 g Dietary Fiber   159 mg Sodium   16 mg Cholesterol

Chocolate Peanut Butter Brownies

16 brownies

These are the chewiest of all the brownies in this book. It's the peanut butter that makes them so rich and chewy. Kids will love these, and will never guess that they are lower in fat and calories.

Ingredients

2 ounces (2 squares) unsweetened chocolate

1/4 cup plus 1 tablespoon dark corn syrup

1 tablespoon water

3/4 cup all-purpose flour

1 tablespoon unsweetened cocoa

1/2 teaspoon salt

1/4 teaspoon baking soda

3/4 cup granulated sugar

1/4 cup reduced-fat peanut butter

2 large egg whites, at room temperature

1 tablespoon vanilla extract

Preheat oven to 350 degrees F. Lightly coat an 8 × 8 × 2-inch baking pan with vegetable or canola oil spray. In a small saucepan combine chocolate, corn syrup, and water. Melt over low heat, stirring until smooth. Remove from heat and cool for 10 minutes.

In a small bowl combine flour, cocoa, salt, and baking soda. In a medium-size mixing bowl combine sugar, peanut butter, egg whites, vanilla, and cooled chocolate mixture. Beat on low speed of electric mixer until creamy. Stir in the dry ingredients to make a smooth batter. Pour into prepared pan.

Bake for approximately 18 to 20 minutes. These brownies are supposed to be chewy and moist, so underbaking them a little is better than overbaking them. When done they should be slightly firm to the touch. Cool completely in pan, on a rack, before cutting into 16 squares using the hot-knife method described in General Baking Tips. Store in an airtight container.

Each serving provides

121 Calories   26% Calories from Fat   4 g Fat
21 g Carbohydrates   3 g Protein   5 mg Calcium
1 g Dietary Fiber   162 mg Sodium   0 mg Cholesterol

Fudgy Brownies

16 brownies

These brownies are made with an extra ounce of chocolate for that moist, fudgy texture—perfect for those midnight chocolate cravings!

Ingredients

3 ounces (3 squares) unsweetened chocolate

2 tablespoons brewed black coffee

1/4 cup plus 1 tablespoon dark corn syrup

3/4 cup all-purpose flour

3/4 teaspoon salt

1/4 teaspoon baking soda

3/4 cup granulated sugar

1/3 cup fat-free ricotta cheese

1 large whole egg plus 1 large egg white, at room temperature

1 tablespoon vanilla extract

Preheat oven to 350 degrees F. Lightly coat an 8 × 8 × 2-inch baking pan with vegetable or canola oil spray. In a small saucepan combine chocolate, coffee, and corn syrup. Melt over low heat, stirring until smooth. Remove from heat and cool for 10 minutes.

Combine flour, salt, and baking soda. In a medium-size bowl combine sugar, ricotta, whole egg, egg white, and vanilla. Whisk together until smooth. Whisk in the cooled chocolate mixture. Stir in the dry ingredients to make a smooth batter and pour into prepared pan.

Bake for approximately 18 to 20 minutes. When done, cake should indent slightly in the center when touched, but should not be firm. These are very moist brownies and are better off if they are a little bit underbaked as opposed to overbaked. Cool completely in pan, on a rack, before cutting into 16 squares, using the hot-knife method described in General Baking Tips. Store in an airtight container.

Each serving provides

112 Calories   26% Calories from Fat   3 g Fat
20 g Carbohydrates   3 g Protein   21 mg Calcium
0 g Dietary Fiber   147 mg Sodium   14 mg Cholesterol

Turtle Brownies

16 brownies

Have you ever had a turtle? It is an incredible candy composed of gooey caramel, crunchy pecans, and rich chocolate. Since turtles are my favorite candy, I had no choice but to model a brownie after them.

Ingredients

3 ounces (3 squares) unsweetened chocolate

2 tablespoons brewed black coffee

1/4 cup plus 1 tablespoon dark corn syrup

3/4 cup all-purpose flour

1/4 teaspoon baking soda

3/4 teaspoon salt

3/4 cup granulated sugar

1/3 cup fat-free ricotta cheese

1 large whole egg plus 1 large egg white, at room temperature

1 tablespoon vanilla extract

1/3 cup (approximately 1 1/4 ounces) toasted chopped pecans

3 tablespoons Gooey Caramel Sauce (page 198)

Preheat oven to 350 degrees F. Lightly coat an 8 × 8 × 2-inch baking pan with vegetable or canola oil spray. In a small saucepan combine chocolate, coffee, and corn syrup. Melt over low heat, stirring until smooth. Remove from heat and cool for 10 minutes.

Combine flour, baking soda, and salt. In a medium-size mixing bowl combine sugar, ricotta, whole egg, egg white, and vanilla. Whisk together until smooth. Whisk in the cooled chocolate mixture. Stir in the dry ingredients to make a smooth batter and pour into prepared pan.

Sweet Deceptions

Sprinkle the toasted pecans all over the surface of the batter and drizzle the caramel over the pecans. Bake for 18 to 20 minutes. These are very soft and gooey on top because of the caramel and I don't recommend touching the center for doneness. Use your best judgment, but they will be even better if they are slightly under-done as they are meant to be soft, fudgy, and gooey. Cool completely in pan, on a rack, before cutting into 16 squares using the hot-knife method described in General Baking Tips.

Each serving provides

137 Calories   32% Calories from Fat   5 g Fat
23 g Carbohydrates   3 g Protein   22 mg Calcium
1 g Dietary Fiber   164 mg Sodium   14 mg Cholesterol

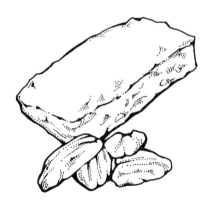

Apple Raisin Oatmeal Bars

20 bars

These treats are great to individually wrap and stuff into back-packs, or take along on bike rides. They work well as an energy bar for all kinds of activities.

Ingredients

2 1/2 cups all-purpose flour
2 1/2 cups old-fashioned oats
1/2 teaspoon salt
1 teaspoon baking soda
1/2 cup chopped raisins or sultanas
1 teaspoon ground allspice
1 teaspoon ground ginger
1 teaspoon ground cloves
1 cup firmly packed brown sugar
1/2 cup granulated sugar

1/4 cup (1/2 stick) light but-ter, at room temperature
1/3 cup honey
1/2 cup lowfat ricotta cheese
1 large whole egg plus 1 egg white, at room temperature
1 tablespoon vanilla extract
1 medium Granny Smith apple, coarsely chopped

Preheat oven to 350 degrees F. Lightly coat a 9 × 13-inch bak-ing pan with nonstick cooking spray and dust with flour. In a large bowl combine flour, oats, salt, baking soda, chopped raisins, and spices. Remove core from apple, quarter it and chop in a food processor until coarse but not pureed. Set chopped apple aside.

In a large bowl cream both sugars, butter, and honey on the medium speed of electric mixer until smooth. Beat in ricotta, whole egg, egg white, and vanilla. Stir in the chopped apple and then the dry ingredients. Spread evenly in prepared pan using a rubber spatula.

Sweet Deceptions

Bake for 25 to 30 minutes, until light golden brown and slightly firm to the touch. Cool completely in pan before cutting into bars. To cut into 20 bars, first cut down the middle lengthwise and cut each half into 10 bars. Store in an airtight container.

Each serving provides

222 Calories   12% Calories from Fat   3 g Fat
45 g Carbohydrates   5 g Protein   55 mg Calcium
2 g Dietary Fiber   140 mg Sodium   17 mg Cholesterol

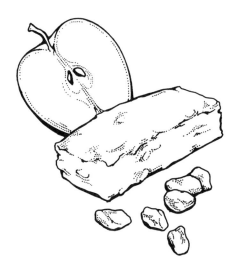

Carrot Cake Squares with Cream Cheese Frosting

24 squares

Making lowfat carrot cake that is actually worth eating is no easy task. It usually has a very large amount of oil in it, which is probably why it tastes so good! I may have lowered the fat content in these squares, but you'll find no skimping when it comes to the cream cheese frosting!

For the cake:

2 cups all-purpose flour	1 tablespoon canola oil
1/2 cup whole wheat flour	1/2 cup lowfat ricotta cheese
2 teaspoons baking powder	
1 teaspoon baking soda	3 large egg whites, at room temperature
1 teaspoon salt	
1 teaspoon ground ginger	1/4 cup dark corn syrup
1/2 teaspoon ground allspice	1 cup firmly packed brown sugar
1/4 teaspoon ground cloves	1 1/3 cups grated carrots (about 3 medium-size carrots)
1/4 teaspoon ground cinnamon	
1/2 cup lowfat buttermilk	1/2 cup chopped raisins or sultanas
1/4 cup orange juice	

For the cream cheese frosting:

1/2 cup plus 2 tablespoons (6 ounces) fat-free cream cheese, at room temperature	3 tablespoons light butter, at room temperature
	1/2 teaspoon vanilla extract
1/2 cup (4 ounces) light Neufchâtel cheese, at room temperature	1 teaspoon grated lemon peel
	2 teaspoons fresh lemon juice
1/2 cup powdered sugar, sifted	

Preheat oven to 350 degrees F. Lightly coat a 9 × 13-inch baking pan with vegetable or canola oil spray and dust with flour. In a medium-size bowl combine both flours, baking powder, baking soda, salt, and spices.

In a large bowl combine buttermilk, orange juice, oil, ricotta, egg whites, corn syrup, and brown sugar. Whisk together until smooth. Stir in grated carrots and chopped raisins. Mix in dry ingredients until thoroughly combined and pour into prepared pan.

Bake for 30 to 40 minutes, or until a cake tester inserted into the center comes out clean. Cool completely in pan before icing.

To make the frosting, combine all frosting ingredients in a medium-size bowl and beat on medium speed of electric mixer until smooth and creamy. Spread evenly over cooled cake and cut into 24 squares using the hot-knife method described in General Baking Tips. Store in an airtight container.

Each serving provides

147 Calories   19% Calories from Fat   3 g Fat
26 g Carbohydrates   5 g Protein   80 mg Calcium
1 g Dietary Fiber   255 mg Sodium   10 mg Cholesterol

Caramel Coconut Bars

24 bars

These bars have a taste and texture quite similar to pecan pie, only I have used coconut instead of pecans. They are wonderful with afternoon coffee or tea.

For the crust:

1 3/4 cups all-purpose flour
 3/4 teaspoon baking soda
 1/4 teaspoon salt
 1/2 cup firmly packed
    brown sugar
   2 tablespoons granulated
    sugar
 1/3 cup light butter, at room
    temperature

   2 teaspoons light corn
    syrup
   1 large egg white, at room
    temperature
   1 teaspoon vanilla extract
 1/3 cup lowfat ricotta
    cheese

For the topping:

 3/4 cup firmly packed
    brown sugar
   1 cup light corn syrup
   3 large egg whites, at
    room temperature
1 1/2 teaspoons salt

   1 tablespoon vanilla
    extract
   2 tablespoons all-purpose
    flour
 3/4 cup lightly toasted,
    sweetened, flaked
    coconut

Preheat oven to 350 degrees F. Lightly coat a 9 × 13-inch baking pan with vegetable or canola oil spray and dust with flour. To prepare crust, in a small bowl combine flour, baking soda, and salt.

In a medium-size mixing bowl cream both sugars, butter, and corn syrup on medium speed of electric mixer until smooth. Beat in egg white, vanilla, and ricotta. Stir in the dry ingredients to make a soft dough.

Transfer dough to prepared baking pan and, using floured hands, press evenly into the bottom of the pan. Set aside while you prepare the topping.

In a medium-size bowl combine brown sugar, corn syrup, egg whites, salt, vanilla, and flour. Whisk together until smooth. Stir in toasted coconut.

Pour topping over prepared crust and bake for 20 to 30 minutes. Topping should be set and light golden brown. Cool completely in pan before cutting into 24 bars using the hot-knife method described in General Baking Tips. To cut into 24 bars, first cut down the middle lengthwise and then cut each half into 12 bars. Store in an airtight container.

Each serving provides

160 Calories   15% Calories from Fat   3 g Fat
32 g Carbohydrates   2 g Protein   32 mg Calcium
1 g Dietary Fiber   246 mg Sodium   6 mg Cholesterol

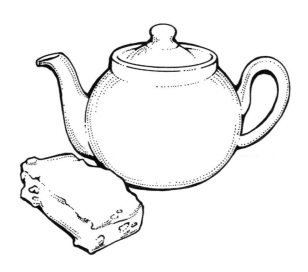

Cookies, Bars, and Squares

Key Lime Squares

Key lime pie is named after the exceptional Florida key limes. They are more tart than regular limes. However, they are not easy to come by unless you live in Florida or the Caribbean. Regular limes will work just as well for these refreshing little squares. These delights are great to serve with any kind of spicy food.

For the crust:

1¼ cups all-purpose flour
⅓ cup powdered sugar
¼ teaspoon baking soda

¼ teaspoon salt
½ cup (1 stick) light butter, at room temperature

For the filling:

1 large whole egg plus 2 large egg whites, at room temperature
1 cup granulated sugar
1 tablespoon grated lime peel

¼ cup fresh lime juice
1½ teaspoons cornstarch
¼ cup toasted, sweetened, flaked coconut

Preheat oven to 350 degrees F. Lightly coat an 8 × 8 × 2-inch baking pan with vegetable or canola oil spray and dust with flour. To prepare the crust, in a medium-size bowl combine flour, sugar, baking soda, salt, and butter. It is easiest to mix this dough using a stand mixer with a paddle attachment, but if you don't have one you can mix it by hand just as successfully. Work the ingredients together with your fingers until they form a uniform dough.

Press dough evenly into the bottom of prepared pan, pressing it all the way to the edges. Prick the crust a few times with a toothpick and bake for 10 minutes. While the crust is baking, prepare the filling.

In a medium-size bowl combine whole egg, egg whites, and sugar. Whisk together until smooth, then whisk in lime peel, lime juice, and cornstarch until mixture is smooth and cornstarch is dissolved. When crust has baked for 10 minutes, pour lime mixture over hot crust and return to oven for an additional 10 to 15 minutes or until topping is set. Cool in pan completely. Sprinkle the top with the toasted coconut and cut into 16 squares using the hot-knife method described in General Baking Tips. Store in an airtight container in the refrigerator.

Each serving provides

132 Calories   28% Calories from Fat   4 g Fat
23 g Carbohydrates   2 g Protein   4 mg Calcium
0 g Dietary Fiber   107 mg Sodium   23 mg Cholesterol

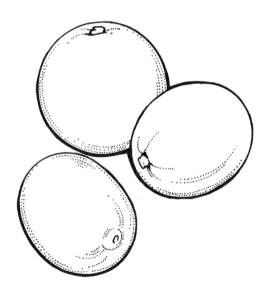

Cookies, Bars, and Squares

Luscious Lemon Squares

These treats are my lowfat version of the classic lemon bar, and no dessert book would be complete without a recipe for them. They are ever-so-delicate and refreshing, especially in the summer when you want something sweet but not too heavy.

For the crust:

1 1/4 cups all-purpose flour	1/4 teaspoon salt
1/3 cup powdered sugar	1/2 cup (1 stick) light butter, at room temperature
1/4 teaspoon baking soda	

For the filling:

1 large whole egg plus 2 large egg whites, at room temperature	1 tablespoon grated lemon peel
1 cup granulated sugar	1/4 cup fresh lemon juice
	1 1/2 teaspoons cornstarch

Preheat oven to 350 degrees F. Lightly coat an 8 × 8 × 2-inch baking pan with vegetable or canola oil spray and dust with flour. To prepare crust, in a medium-size bowl combine flour, sugar, baking soda, salt, and butter. It is easiest to mix this dough using a stand mixer with the paddle attachment, but if you don't have one you can mix it just as successfully by hand. Work the ingredients together with your fingers until they become a uniform dough.

Press dough evenly into the bottom of prepared pan, pressing it all the way to the edges. Prick the crust a few times with a toothpick and bake for 10 minutes. While the crust is baking, prepare the filling.

In a medium-size bowl combine whole egg, egg whites, and sugar. Whisk together until smooth. Whisk in lemon peel, lemon juice, and cornstarch until mixture is smooth and cornstarch has dissolved. When crust has baked for 10 minutes, pour lemon mixture over hot crust and return to oven for an additional 10 to 15 minutes, or until topping is set. Cool in pan completely before cutting into 16 squares using the hot-knife method described in General Baking Tips. Store in an airtight container in the refrigerator.

Serving Suggestion

For an added touch, these look really nice with a dusting of powdered sugar.

Each serving provides

123 Calories   25% Calories from Fat   3 g Fat
22 g Carbohydrates   2 g Protein   4 mg Calcium
0 g Dietary Fiber   102 mg Sodium   23 mg Cholesterol

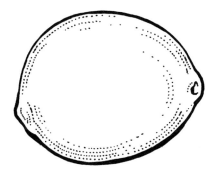

Peanut Butter Cookies

60 cookies

Ingredients

1 1/4 cups all-purpose flour
1/2 cup whole wheat flour
1/2 teaspoon baking soda
1/2 cup firmly packed brown sugar
1/2 cup granulated sugar plus 1/3 cup granulated sugar for rolling cookies

6 tablespoons (3/4 stick) light butter, at room temperature
1 cup reduced-fat peanut butter
2 large egg whites, at room temperature
2 teaspoons vanilla extract

Preheat oven to 350 degrees F. Line a cookie sheet with foil or parchment paper. In a small bowl combine both flours and baking soda.

In a large mixing bowl cream brown sugar, 1/2 cup granulated sugar, butter, and peanut butter on medium speed of electric mixer until smooth. Beat in egg whites and vanilla until fully incorporated. Stir in dry ingredients to make a soft dough.

Roll dough into 1-inch balls, roll in sugar, and place 2 1/2 inches apart on prepared cookie sheet. Use a fork to crisscross and flatten each cookie.

Bake for 10 to 12 minutes or until light golden brown. Cool completely on a rack and store in an airtight container.

Each serving provides

61 Calories   33% Calories from Fat   2 g Fat
9 g Carbohydrates   2 g Protein   2 mg Calcium
0 g Dietary Fiber   47 mg Sodium   2 mg Cholesterol

Custards, Mousses, and Decadent Creations

Banana and Chocolate Chip Bread Pudding

Banana Flan

Caramel Apple and Walnut Cobbler

Cherry Almond Bread Pudding

Classic Chocolate Mousse

Crème Brûlée with Spiced Rum

Crème Caramel

Devil's Food Pots de Crème

Frozen Coffee Cream

Frozen Toasted-Almond Mousse Cake

Lemon Apricot Pudding Cakes with Blueberry Sauce

Lemon Ginger Mousse

Macadamia Praline Mousse

Tiramisù

Peach Blueberry Cobbler with Cornmeal Crisp

Sierra Mud Slide Pie

Chapter Five

Custards, Mousses, and Decadent Creations

Creamy custards and dreamy mousses that are light as a feather fill this chapter and you'll find the true meaning of the word *decadence*, from Tiramisù to Crème Brûlée complete with a crackly sugar crust. The only thing you'll be missing is the catastrophic amount of fat that usually accompany these types of desserts. I have compiled a selection of classic favorites combined with some fabulous new creations, such as Sierra Mud Slide Pie and Frozen Coffee Cream. The following tips will help you with the techniques in this chapter.

Custards

Once you know the secrets for custard-making success, you'll find yourself making them more often. For some, the idea of making custard is intimidating—so many things can go wrong, from scorching it on the stove to curdling it in the oven. It's all a matter of giving the custard extra attention. You always have to keep an eye on how it looks at certain stages of the cooking process.

The most important thing to keep in mind is the delicacy of the eggs. If cooked too long, the custard will curdle. Even a properly cooked custard will continue to cook a bit as it cools, and can still curdle. Cooling custards and custard sauces over ice water halts the cooking process and quickly lowers their temperature. Baked custards require a different technique than most other desserts. To prevent scorching and curdling, they are baked in a water bath at a lower temperature than most other desserts. In other words, they are slow-cooked.

For baking custards, 300 to 325 degrees Fahrenheit is the optimal temperature range. The most effective pan to use for the water bath is a large glass baking dish, 3 to 4 inches deep, or a roasting pan with the same depth. There should be enough room in the pan for all of the custard cups, with room to spare between them so that they do not touch. Hot water is poured around the cups to reach three quarters of the way up their sides. The water bath acts as a kind of insulation for the custards and helps to control the amount of heat that reaches them.

Once the cups are in the pan and the water has been poured in, it can be quite a trick to maneuver it to the oven. If the pan tips too much one way or the other, you will end up with water in your custards, and they will be ruined. I find it best to place the pan with the cups in the oven first, then pour in the hot water. When it comes to removing them, it is pretty much your call. There won't be as much water in the pan due to evaporation, and a steady hand should have no troubles. If you don't want to take any chances,

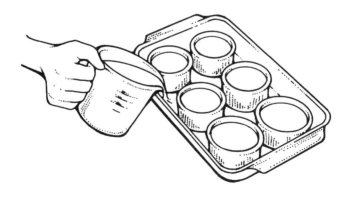

simply remove some of the water first. You can do this easily with a small ladle or even a turkey baster.

When baking custards, it is not always so easy to tell when they are done. It takes practice. You will learn to judge the stage of doneness simply by giving one of the cups a slight jiggle. If the custard is firm, it is done and should be removed from the oven. I have found that it isn't necessary to cook custards all the way to the firm stage; in fact, they will more likely have the best texture if they move ever so slightly in the center when you jiggle them. They should not be liquid in the center. (This method does not apply to custards that are baked in a tart shell.) When they reach this stage, you can remove them from the oven. As they cool in the water bath, they will continue to cook just enough to achieve that perfect custard texture. When the cups are cool enough to handle, remove them from the water.

When storing the custards in the refrigerator, be sure to keep them tightly covered with plastic wrap to keep them from drying out and from absorbing any refrigerator odors.

Mousses

You will find several recipes here for mousse, from Classic Chocolate Mousse served from an elegant glass, to frozen mousse cakes that are reminiscent of eating the richest ice cream. These desserts aren't at all difficult to make; however, a gorgeous texture is crucial for their success. It's all in the folding! Use a delicate hand to preserve those precious air pockets you've made! Always use a rubber spatula to fold the beaten egg whites and/or whipped topping into the mousse base. The whole trick here is to fold as little as possible with great efficiency. Yes, this can be done! Go for a rolling motion with the spatula, bringing the mixture up from the bottom of the bowl and rotating the bowl with each stroke of the spatula. Go down through the center of the mousse and surface on the edge. Fold only until there are no streaks showing in the mousse. Never stir it or beat it, as this deflates the mousse, breaking down those tiny air pockets that are responsible for its

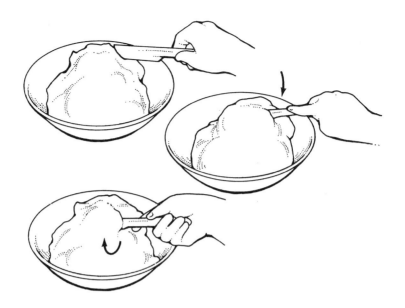

wonderful texture. Practice does make perfect, and you can practice folding with a bowl of beaten egg whites just to help you feel more comfortable with the motions.

When the mousse has been folded to perfection, you have the option of chilling it in a large bowl and dishing it up later, or spooning it into fancy glasses or dessert cups and chilling them individually. As with the custards, keep them tightly covered with plastic wrap in the refrigerator.

Sweet Deceptions

Banana and Chocolate Chip Bread Pudding

12 servings

Ingredients

8 cups soft French bread (approximately 1 large loaf), cut into 1-inch cubes, crust included

4 large whole eggs

3/4 cup granulated sugar

1 tablespoon vanilla extract

1 large banana, very ripe

3/4 cup liquid nondairy creamer

1/2 cup light nondairy creamer

1/4 cup granulated sugar

Preheat oven to 350 degrees F. Lightly coat an 8-inch square baking pan with vegetable or canola oil spray. Put the bread cubes in a large mixing bowl.

In a medium-size bowl combine eggs, 3/4 cup sugar, and vanilla. Whisk together until smooth. In a food processor fitted with the metal blade, puree banana and regular creamer. Whisk in to the egg mixture. Whisk in light creamer until smooth. Pour custard over bread and toss well, letting the bread absorb the liquid. Toss in the chocolate chips. Pour into prepared baking dish and use the back of a large spoon or a spatula to press mixture down and compact it, so that the top is even and there are no holes in the pudding. Sprinkle surface with the remaining 1/4 cup sugar.

Bake for approximately 30 to 40 minutes. Pudding should spring back when you touch it, and should be very lightly browned on top. Cool on a rack. You can serve pudding warm or cold. Store in an airtight container in the refrigerator.

Serving Suggestions

I love to serve this pudding warm on a pool of warm Chocolate Sauce (page 201), and maybe a dollop of light whipped topping. Gooey Caramel Sauce (page 198) is also a decadent addition.

Each serving provides

227 Calories   26% Calories from Fat   7 g Fat
37 g Carbohydrates   5 g Protein   38 mg Calcium
1 g Dietary Fiber   172 mg Sodium   70 mg Cholesterol

Banana Flan

If you're a fan of custards like I am, then you're sure to enjoy this twist on the classic Crème Caramel. The addition of a very ripe banana makes the custard rich and creamy.

For caramel:

3/4 cup granulated sugar | 1/3 cup water

For custard:

1/2 cup granulated sugar
3 large whole eggs plus
   2 large egg whites, at
   room temperature
2 teaspoons vanilla extract
1 cup evaporated skim milk

1/4 cup light sour cream
1/4 cup liquid nondairy
   creamer
1 tablespoon cornstarch
1 medium, very ripe banana,
   mashed (about 1/2 cup)

Preheat oven to 325 degrees F. You will need six 5-ounce ramekins. Place them in a shallow baking dish or roasting pan, leaving space between them.

To prepare caramel for bottom of cups, in a small saucepan combine the 3/4 cup sugar and water. Cook over high heat, undisturbed, until sugar begins to turn light amber in color. As soon as the sugar is getting close to a golden amber, take the pan off the heat and let it continue to caramelize to a deep golden amber, swirling the pan to even out the color. Once the sugar is a deep golden amber, pour approximately 1 tablespoon of the caramel into the bottom of each ramekin. Swirl each ramekin to disperse the caramel evenly over the bottom. Set aside to cool, and discard excess caramel.

To prepare the custard, in a medium-size bowl whisk together the 1/2 cup sugar, whole eggs, egg whites, and vanilla. Whisk in the evaporated milk. In a food processor fitted with the metal blade, puree the sour cream, liquid creamer, cornstarch, and mashed banana. Add to the egg mixture and whisk together until smooth.

122   Sweet Deceptions

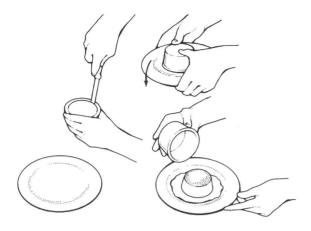

Strain mixture through a fine-mesh sieve. Divide custard evenly among the 6 ramekins. Pour in enough hot water to reach three quarters of the way up the sides of the ramekins.

Bake for approximately 45 minutes to 1 hour. The centers of custards should jiggle ever so slightly, but should not be liquid. Cool custards to room temperature in the pan, then remove them from their water bath and refrigerate for at least 4 hours or overnight before serving.

To unmold and serve custards, run a sharp paring knife around the edge of each custard and invert the ramekin onto a serving plate. Using your thumbs, hold the ramekin tight to the plate and give both plate and ramekin a strong downward shake which will release the custard from the mold. You may have to try a few times, but you will know when you've succeeded because you will hear the custard plop onto the plate. Lift off the ramekin, garnish, and serve.

Serving Suggestions

Whenever I make flan of any kind, I always pour extra Gem Caramel Sauce (page 200) on them because there never seems to be enough sauce when they're unmolded. Light whipped topping complements them wonderfully, and since we are talking about banana here, I think some chocolate sauce drizzled over it would be quite appropriate!

Each serving provides

273 Calories   13% Calories from Fat   4 g Fat
52 g Carbohydrates   8 g Protein   146 mg Calcium
0 g Dietary Fiber   107 mg Sodium   110 mg Cholesterol

Custards, Mousses, and Decadent Creations

Caramel Apple and Walnut Cobbler

This dessert is perfect for serving on those cold winter nights during the holidays! Tender Granny Smith apples are quickly stewed with a light caramel flavor, and topped with a fluffy toasted walnut scone.

For caramel apple filling:

- 1 tablespoon cornstarch
- 2 teaspoons vanilla extract
- 1½ tablespoons water

- ¼ cup water
- ⅓ cup firmly packed brown sugar

- ⅓ cup granulated sugar
- 1 tablespoon light butter
- ¼ teaspoon salt
- 6 medium Granny Smith apples, quartered and cut in ¼-inch slices

For walnut scone topping:

- 1½ cups all-purpose flour
- ¼ teaspoon salt
- ½ teaspoon ground cinnamon
- 2½ teaspoons baking powder
- 2 tablespoons granulated sugar
- 2 tablespoons butter-flavored shortening

- ⅓ cup chopped walnuts, lightly toasted
- ¾ cup lowfat buttermilk
- 1 large egg white, at room temperature
- 1 tablespoon vanilla extract
- 2 tablespoons granulated sugar

You will need an 8 × 8 × 2-inch baking pan. To make the caramel apple filling, in a small bowl combine the cornstarch, vanilla, and the 1¹/₂ tablespoons water.

In a deep, heavy-bottomed skillet, combine the ¹/₄ cup water, both sugars, butter, and salt. Cook over high heat until mixture is bubbly and thick, approximately 2 to 3 minutes, stirring occasionally with a wooden spoon. Add the sliced apples and cook for approximately 5 minutes, or until apples are tender but not mushy. Add the cornstarch mixture, stirring to distribute, and continue to cook for 1 more minute, until mixture thickens. Pour into pan and pat level. Set aside to prepare topping.

Preheat oven to 375 degrees F. In a large bowl combine flour, salt, cinnamon, baking powder, and 2 tablespoons sugar. Add the shortening and rub the mixture together with your fingers to completely distribute the shortening. Mixture will be coarse. Add toasted walnuts and toss to combine.

In a small bowl combine buttermilk, egg white, and vanilla and whisk together until smooth. Pour into dry ingredients and mix with a fork to form a soft dough. Use a large spoon or a spatula to cover the entire surface of the apples with dollops of the dough. It should look rough and bumpy, and a few small gaps here and there are okay. Sprinkle the surface of the dough with the remaining 2 tablespoons sugar.

Bake for approximately 20 minutes, or until light golden brown and filling is bubbly around the edges. Cool on a rack for at least 1 hour before serving. Store in the refrigerator, covered with plastic wrap.

Serving Suggestions

I would definitely serve this dessert warm and à la mode with Gooey Caramel Sauce (page 198). It is also delicious with a dollop of light whipped topping.

Each serving provides

271 Calories   18% Calories from Fat   5 g Fat
53 g Carbohydrates   4 g Protein   58 mg Calcium
2 g Dietary Fiber   240 mg Sodium   1 mg Cholesterol

Cherry Almond Bread Pudding

12 servings

Don't restrict this bread pudding to after-dinner dessert—I find it perfect for breakfast, as it slices so nicely and goes beautifully with coffee.

Ingredients

8 cups (approximately 1 large loaf) soft French bread, cut into 1-inch cubes, crust included

4 large whole eggs

3/4 cup granulated sugar

2 teaspoons vanilla extract

1 teaspoon almond extract

3/4 cups liquid nondairy creamer

1/2 cup light liquid nondairy creamer

1 1/4 cups (10 ounces) cherry pie filling

1/4 cup granulated sugar

Preheat oven to 350 degrees F. Lightly coat an 8-inch square baking pan with vegetable or canola oil spray. Put the bread cubes in a large mixing bowl.

In a medium-size bowl combine eggs and 3/4 cup sugar and whisk together until smooth. Whisk in the vanilla, almond extract, regular creamer, and light creamer until smooth. Stir in 1 cup of the cherry pie filling, reserving 1/4 cup for the top of pudding. Pour custard over bread and toss well, so bread absorbs the liquid. Pour into prepared baking dish. Use the back of a large spoon or a spatula to press mixture down and compact it so that the top is even and there are no holes in the pudding. Dot the surface with the reserved 1/4 cup cherries and sprinkle with remaining 1/4 cup sugar.

Bake for approximately 30 to 40 minutes. Pudding should spring back when you touch it, and should be very lightly browned on top. Cool on a rack. You can serve pudding warm or cold. Store in an airtight container in the refrigerator.

Serving Suggestions

This dessert looks very nice when dusted with powdered sugar. A dollop of light whipped topping or a scoop of frozen yogurt adds the perfect touch. You can also serve it on a pool of Crème Anglaise (page 000) with toasted sliced almonds.

Each serving provides

166 Calories   21% Calories from Fat   4 g Fat
26 g Carbohydrates   4 g Protein   35 mg Calcium
3 g Dietary Fiber   171 mg Sodium   70 mg Cholesterol

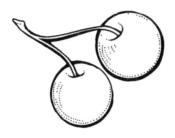

Classic Chocolate Mousse

6 servings

Ingredients

1/4 cup liquid nondairy creamer
1 teaspoon instant coffee crystals
1/4 teaspoon salt
1 ounce (1 square) unsweetened chocolate, chopped
1/2 cup semisweet chocolate chips

1/2 cup (4 ounces) fat-free cream cheese, at room temperature
2 tablespoons unsweetened cocoa
1 tablespoon whiskey
2 teaspoons vanilla extract
3 large egg whites, at room temperature
1/2 cup granulated sugar

In a small saucepan combine creamer, coffee, salt, unsweetened chocolate, and chocolate chips. Place over low heat and stir until melted and smooth. Remove from heat and cool for 10 minutes.

In a food processor fitted with the metal blade, puree cream cheese, cocoa, whiskey, and vanilla. Add the cooled chocolate mixture and process until smooth. Transfer mixture to a large mixing bowl.

In a separate medium-size mixing bowl that is clean and grease-free, beat the egg whites on medium speed of electric mixer until soft peaks form. Increase speed to high and sprinkle in the sugar a tablespoon at a time, beating until all the sugar has been incorporated and egg whites are stiff and glossy. Carefully fold beaten egg whites into chocolate mixture, using a rubber spatula. You can divide mousse between 6 individual cups or glasses, or you can chill it as a whole in a large bowl or soufflé dish. Refrigerate for at least 6 hours or overnight before serving.

This mousse is delicious when served with a dollop of light whipped topping. You can also add some fresh berries or Chocolate Curls (page 192) for an elegant finishing touch.

Each serving provides

208 Calories   38% Calories from Fat   8 g Fat
29 g Carbohydrates   6 g Protein   80 mg Calcium
1 g Dietary Fiber   238 mg Sodium   3 mg Cholesterol

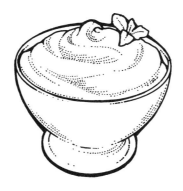

Crème Brûlée with Spiced Rum

6 servings

This dessert is an old favorite that many people have great difficulty saying no to. We're talking about some pretty heavenly stuff, but each little dish will set you back to the tune of almost 500 calories and 45 grams of fat! You'll find a dramatic difference in calories and fat grams between a traditional crème brûlée and my lightened recipe. This version of that divine custard is quite a bit lower in fat but every bit as creamy and delicious, right down to the caramelized sugar crust.

For custard:

2 cups liquid nondairy creamer	1/8 teaspoon salt
1 tablespoon cornstarch	2 teaspoons vanilla extract
2 teaspoons all-purpose flour	2 tablespoons spiced rum (you can use regular rum if you cannot find spiced rum)
1/2 cup granulated sugar	
1 large whole egg plus 3 large egg yolks	1/2 cup sweetened condensed lowfat milk

Burnt sugar topping:

1 tablespoon brown sugar	3 tablespoons granulated sugar

Preheat oven to 325 degrees F. You will need six 5-ounce ramekins. Place them in a shallow baking dish or roasting pan, leaving space between them.

In a small saucepan combine creamer, cornstarch, and flour and whisk together until dissolved. Cook over medium-high heat, stirring constantly with a wooden spoon to prevent scorching, until mixture thickens and coats the back of the spoon. It should be the consistency of heavy cream. Remove from heat and cool for 10 minutes.

In a medium-size bowl combine sugar, whole egg, egg yolks, salt, vanilla, and rum. Whisk together until smooth, then whisk in the condensed milk and cooled creamer mixture. Be careful not to over-whisk as this will create too much foam on the surface of the custards. Strain mixture through a fine-mesh sieve. Divide mixture evenly among the six ramekins and pour enough hot water around them to come three quarters of the way up their sides.

Bake for approximately 45 minutes to 1 hour, or until custards are set. Cool custards to room temperature in the pan, then remove them from their water bath and refrigerate for at least 4 hours or overnight before making burnt sugar topping.

The sugar isn't actually burned but rather caramelized to a golden amber on top of the custard. As it cools, the caramel hardens, making the signature crisp sugar crust.

Preheat broiler. Combine the two sugars, breaking up any lumps. Sprinkle the top of each custard with 2 teaspoons of sugar mixture, spreading it as evenly as possible. Place custards under the broiler until sugar caramelizes to a golden amber. It is best to do only a couple at a time, making it easier to watch them so that the sugar doesn't burn. Refrigerate custards for 1 hour before serving, to harden the sugar crust and cool the custard.

Serving Suggestions

I don't usually serve anything with Crème Brûlée other than a garnish of mint. If you want to jazz it up a bit, fresh berries make a wonderful addition.

Each serving provides

310 Calories   20% Calories from Fat   7 g Fat
49 g Carbohydrates   5 g Protein   78 mg Calcium
0 g Dietary Fiber   148 mg Sodium   36 mg Cholesterol

Crème Caramel

6 servings

This is a lower-fat version of the classic flan. If I see this dessert on the menu, I usually order it. Crème caramel is the perfect end to any meal, especially after a heavy one, because it is such a light and delicate dessert.

For caramel:

3/4 cup granulated sugar | 1/3 cup water

For custard:

3/4 cup granulated sugar	3/4 cup evaporated skim milk
3 large whole eggs plus	3/4 cup liquid nondairy
3 large egg whites, at	creamer
room temperature	1/2 cup light sour cream
1 tablespoon vanilla extract	2 teaspoons cornstarsh

Preheat oven to 325 degrees F. You will need six 5-ounce ramekins. Place them in a shallow baking dish or roasting pan, leaving space between them. To prepare caramel for the bottom of the cups, in a small saucepan combine sugar and water. Cook over high heat, undisturbed, until sugar begins to turn light amber in color. As soon as the sugar is getting close to a golden amber, take the pan off the heat and let it continue to caramelize to a deep golden amber, swirling the pan to even out the color. Once the sugar is deep golden amber, pour approximately 1 tablespoon of the caramel into the bottom of each ramekin. Swirl each ramekin to disperse the caramel evenly over the bottom. Set aside to cool, and discard excess caramel.

To prepare custard, in a medium-size bowl combine the sugar, whole eggs, egg whites, and vanilla, and whisk together until smooth. Whisk in the evaporated milk. In a food processor fitted with the metal blade, puree the creamer, sour cream, and corn-starch. Add to egg mixture and whisk together until smooth. Strain mixture through a fine-mesh sieve. Divide custard evenly among the 6 ramekins. Pour enough hot water around them to come three quarters of the way up their sides.

Bake for approximately 50 minutes to 1 hour, or until a small knife inserted into the center comes out relatively clean and the custards are set. Cool custards to room temperature in the pan, then remove them from their water bath and refrigerate for at least 4 hours or overnight before serving.

To unmold and serve custards, run a sharp paring knife around the edge of each custard and invert the ramekin onto a serving plate (see helpful diagram on page 123). Using your thumbs, hold the ramekin tightly against the plate and give both plate and ramekin a firm downward shake, which will release the custard from the mold. You may have to try a few times, but when you succeed you will hear the custard plop onto the plate. Lift off the ramekin, garnish, and serve.

Serving Suggestions

As with the banana flan, I strongly suggest bathing this custard in extra Gem Caramel Sauce (page 200), as there never seems to be enough sauce after unmolding them. Crème Caramel is also very nice when served with fresh berries and light whipped topping. Don't hesitate to sprinkle some toasted nuts over them.

Each serving provides

325 Calories   20% Calories from Fat   7 g Fat
56 g Carbohydrates   8 g Protein   129 mg Calcium
0 g Dietary Fiber   119 mg Sodium   116 mg Cholesterol

Devil's food Pots de Crème

6 servings

Good things really do come in small packages! These little cups of custard pack a wallop of intense chocolate flavor.

Ingredients

1 cup liquid nondairy creamer

1 1/2 tablespoons dark corn syrup

1 tablespoon cider vinegar

2 ounces (2 squares) unsweetened chocolate, chopped

1/4 cup semisweet chocolate chips

2 large egg yolks plus 1 large whole egg, at room temperature

1 cup granulated sugar

1 tablespoon vanilla extract

2 tablespoons all-purpose flour

2 teaspoons cornstarch

1/2 teaspoon salt

Place six 5-ounce ramekins in a shallow baking dish or roasting pan, leaving space between them. In a small saucepan combine creamer, corn syrup, and vinegar. Place over high heat just until mixture comes to a boil. Remove from heat and add all the chocolate. Stir with a whisk until smooth and chocolate has melted. Set aside to cool.

In a medium-size bowl combine egg yolks, whole egg, sugar, vanilla, flour, cornstarch, and salt. Whisk together until smooth and creamy. Whisk in the cooled chocolate mixture. It may appear slightly separated, but this does not affect the texture of the finished custard. Pour into ramekins, dividing custard evenly among them. Pour enough hot water around the ramekins to come three quarters of the way up their sides. Cover baking dish with foil and bake for approximately 30 minutes, until custards are set. Cool custards to room temperature in the pan, then remove them from their water bath and refrigerate for at least 4 hours or overnight before serving.

Serving Suggestions

These little custards are served right in their ramekins. They are so rich and chocolatey that the only thing they might need is a dollop of light whipped topping.

Each serving provides

320 Calories   37% Calories from Fat   13 g Fat
49 g Carbohydrates   4 g Protein   24 mg Calcium
1 g Dietary Fiber   217 mg Sodium   107 mg Cholesterol

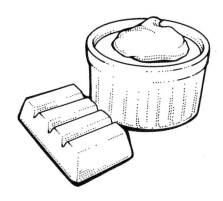

Frozen Coffee Cream

10 to 12 servings

Some days all you want is a scoop of something creamy and frozen, preferably right from the container! If that's the case, you might want to give this recipe a try. I have found it to be the perfect solution to ice cream cravings. Nothing fancy here, just scoop it right out as if it were ice cream. It has a wonderfully creamy coffee flavor and is perfect to scoop into a cone!

Ingredients

2 large egg yolks at room temperature	1/4 cup (2 ounces) light Neufchâtel cheese, at room temperature
1/4 cup granulated sugar	1 tablespoon vanilla extract
1 cup liquid nondairy creamer	1 1/2 tablespoons instant coffee crystals, dissolved in one tablespoon hot water
1 tablespoon all-purpose flour	2 cups light whipped topping
1 tablespoon cornstarch	

In a small saucepan combine egg yolks and sugar and whisk together until creamy. Whisk in the creamer, flour, and cornstarch until dissolved. Place over medium-high heat and cook, stirring constantly with a wooden spoon to prevent scorching, until mixture thickens and coats the back of the spoon. At this point, use the wire whisk again to stir it and smooth out any lumps that may have formed. Remove from heat and stir in the cheese until it is completely melted and mixture is smooth. Whisk in vanilla and coffee.

Place bowl in another bowl filled with ice water and stir until mixture is cool to the touch. Discard ice water. Stir in whipped topping until mixture is smooth and creamy. Pour coffee cream into a shallow 2-quart, freezable container. Freeze overnight.

If you own an ice cream machine, you can double the recipe and freeze it according to the manufacturer's instructions to give the cream even more of an ice cream texture. You can also freeze the cream in individual molds—I like to use tall timbale molds—then dip them in hot water to unmold the frozen cream. They look quite impressive on a pool of custard sauce that has been splashed with other sauces and garnishes.

Serving Suggestions

If you plan to scoop the cream from the container into a dish, I recommend turning it into a sundae, topping it with any of the sauces in Finishing Touches. You can top it off with light whipped topping and nuts, or even Crushed Meringue (page 208).

Each serving provides

96 Calories   58% Calories from Fat   6 g Fat
10 g Carbohydrates   1 g Protein   12 mg Calcium
0 g Dietary Fiber   36 mg Sodium   40 mg Cholesterol

Frozen Toasted-Almond Mousse Cake

12 servings

For cake base:

3/4 cup all-purpose flour
 1   teaspoon baking powder
1/4 teaspoon salt
 1   tablespoon vegetable
     shortening
1/3 cup granulated sugar
 2   tablespoons lowfat ricotta
     cheese

1/3 cup milk (2 percent)
 1   teaspoon vanilla extract

 2   large egg whites, at room
     temperature
 2   tablespoons granulated
     sugar

For mousse:

1/4 cup plus 2 tablespoons
     (3 ounces) light
     Neufchâtel cheese, at
     room temperature
1/2 cup (4 ounces) fat-free
     cream cheese, at room
     temperature
 1   tablespoon vanilla extract
 1   teaspoon almond extract

 1   tablespoon liquid
     nondairy creamer
1/2 cup ground toasted
     almonds
 3   large egg whites, at room
     temperature
1/4 teaspoon cream of tartar
3/4 cup granulated sugar

Preheat oven to 350 degrees F. Lightly coat a 9-inch spring-form pan with vegetable or canola oil spray and dust with flour. In a medium-size bowl combine flour, baking powder, and salt.

In a separate medium-size mixing bowl cream the shortening, sugar, and ricotta on medium speed of electric mixer until creamy. Beat in milk and vanilla, and stir in the dry ingredients.

In a small mixing bowl that is clean and grease-free, beat the egg whites on medium speed of electric mixer until soft peaks form. Increase speed to high and sprinkle in the sugar, beating until firm peaks form. Carefully fold into batter using a rubber spatula. Pour batter into prepared pan and smooth the top with a spatula.

Bake for approximately 20 minutes, or until a cake tester inserted into the center comes out clean. Cool completely in the pan on a rack.

To make the mousse, in a food processor fitted with the metal blade, puree Neufchâtel cheese, cream cheese, vanilla, almond extract, and creamer. Transfer to a medium-size bowl and stir in the toasted almonds.

In a separate medium-size mixing bowl that is clean and grease-free, combine the egg whites with the cream of tartar. Beat on medium speed of electric mixer until soft peaks form. Increase speed to high and sprinkle in the sugar a tablespoon at a time, beating until all of the sugar has been incorporated and meringue is stiff and glossy. Carefully fold meringue into cheese mixture, using a rubber spatula. Pour mousse into the pan over the cake base. Cover with plastic wrap and freeze for at least 6 hours or overnight before serving.

To unmold, run a hot knife all the way around the edge of pan to release the mousse from the sides, and unlatch the pan. Cut into 12 servings using the hot-knife method described in General Baking Tips.

Serving Suggestions

Try serving this mousse cake on caramel and chocolate sauces for the ultimate frozen treat. You can also top it with a few Chocolate Curls (page 191). Serving it on a berry sauce makes an interesting and delicious combination.

Each serving provides

184 Calories   28% Calories from Fat   6 g Fat
27 g Carbohydrates   6 g Protein   79 mg Calcium
1 g Dietary Fiber   198 mg Sodium   11 mg Cholesterol

Lemon Apricot Pudding Cakes
with Blueberry Sauce

6 servings

These little dessert cakes have a moist texture that is a cross between cake and pudding. They have a refreshing flavor of lemon combined with apricot, and are absolutely decadent when served warm, covered in blueberry sauce.

For pudding cakes:

1 cup plus 1 tablespoon all-purpose flour

3 tablespoons cornstarch

1/4 teaspoon salt

3/4 cup granulated sugar

1/4 cup (2 ounces) fat-free cream cheese, at room temperature

1/4 cup Apricot Puree (page 205)

1 large whole egg, at room temperature

1 large egg white, at room temperature

1/2 teaspoon lemon extract

2 tablespoons grated lemon peel

1/4 cup fresh lemon juice

2 large egg whites, at room temperature

1 tablespoon granulated sugar

For blueberry sauce:

2 cups frozen blueberries

2 tablespoons granulated sugar

2 teaspoons cornstarch

3 tablespoons water

Preheat oven to 325 degrees F. Generously coat six 5-ounce pudding molds or ramekins with vegetable shortening, and place them in a shallow baking dish or roasting pan, leaving space between them. To make the pudding cakes, sift together the flour, cornstarch, and salt in a small bowl.

In a food processor fitted with the metal blade, puree the 3/4 cup sugar, cream cheese, and apricot puree. Add whole egg, egg white, lemon extract, lemon peel, and lemon juice. Process again until smooth. Transfer mixture to a large bowl and whisk in the flour mixture, a quarter of a cup at a time, until batter is smooth and uniform.

In a medium-size mixing bowl that is clean and grease-free, beat the egg whites on medium speed of electric mixer until soft peaks form. Sprinkle in the remaining tablespoon of sugar and continue to beat until firm peaks form. Carefully fold beaten egg whites into batter using a rubber spatula. Be careful not to over-fold as the batter will deflate and lose volume. Divide evenly among the 6 prepared molds. Pour enough hot water in pan to come three quarters of the way up to the sides of the ramekins.

Bake for approximately 35 to 40 minutes. Puddings will be firm to the touch in the center. When done, immediately unmold pudding cakes onto a cookie sheet that has been lined with foil and lightly coated with vegetable or canola oil spray. If you baked the cakes in ramekins, you can cool and serve them right in their dishes. Cover unmolded pudding cakes with a sheet of plastic wrap; this helps lock in moisture as they cool. Store in the refrigerator, covered with plastic wrap.

To make the sauce, combine all sauce ingredients in a medium-size saucepan and cook over medium-high heat until sauce thickens. Stir gently to keep from crushing the berries. Store in an airtight container in the refrigerator.

For assembly, transfer unmolded pudding cakes to dessert plates and spoon some blueberry sauce over each one. You can serve these delights either at room temperature or warmed. To warm the cakes, loosely cover them with foil and place in a 325 degree F oven for about 10 minutes.

Serving Suggestions

These desserts are so fresh and simple that the only other garnish I would suggest is a small dollop of light whipped topping and maybe a small mound of Apricot Puree.

Each serving provides

290 Calories   4% Calories from Fat   1 g Fat
64 g Carbohydrates   7 g Protein   48 mg Calcium
2 g Dietary Fiber   188 mg Sodium   38 mg Cholesterol

Custards, Mousses, and Decadent Creations

Lemon Ginger Mousse

6 servings

This mousse may sound very light and non-threatening in the decadence category, but don't let the name fool you! It is light compared to the other desserts, and very refreshing with its tart, lemony taste accented by just the right zestiness from the fresh ginger. However, it hides a decadent, rich texture, and I found myself having to change the number of servings from five to six! Be warned, it has an alluring and addictive flavor, so don't be surprised to find that you can't stop eating it!

Ingredients

1/3 cup granulated sugar
2 large egg yolks, at room temperature
2 tablespoons cornstarch
1 tablespoon grated lemon peel
1/2 cup fresh lemon juice

2 tablespoons grated fresh ginger

3 large egg whites, at room temperature
1/8 teaspoon cream of tartar
1/3 cup granulated sugar
1 cup light whipped topping plus additional for garnish, if desired

In a small bowl whisk together the 1/3 cup sugar, egg yolks, and cornstarch until smooth. Whisk in the lemon peel, lemon juice, and ginger. Pour mixture into a double boiler and cook over medium-high heat, stirring with a whisk, until mixture is very thick. Transfer to a medium-size bowl and cover with a sheet of plastic wrap, pressing it directly against the lemon curd. This step will prevent a skin from forming over the top as it cools. Refrigerate for 1 hour or until cold.

In a separate medium-size bowl that is clean and grease-free, combine egg whites and cream of tartar. Beat on medium speed of electric mixer until soft peaks form. Increase speed to high and sprinkle in the remaining 1/3 cup sugar a tablespoon at a time, beating until all the sugar has been incorporated and the mixture is very firm and glossy. Vigorously stir a quarter of the beaten egg whites into lemon curd to loosen it up. Then carefully fold in remaining egg whites and light whipped topping all at once, using a rubber spatula. Spoon into individual glasses or small bowls, or carefully ladle entire mixture into a large bowl. Refrigerate for 4 hours or overnight before serving.

Serving Suggestions

This mousse looks beautiful when chilled in Champagne flutes. Fresh berries are a perfect accompaniment, along with a small dollop of light whipped topping. For an extra special touch, serve with Sugared Hazelnut Biscuits (page 96).

Each serving provides

151 Calories   26% Calories from Fat   4 g Fat
29 g Carbohydrates   3 g Protein   15 mg Calcium
0 g Dietary Fiber   50 mg Sodium   70 mg Cholesterol

Macadamia Praline Mousse

6 servings

You'll find this mousse to be light as a feather in texture, but sinfully rich and decadent in taste.

For macadamia praline:

4 ounces (about 3/4 cup) unsalted macadamia nuts	1 cup granulated sugar 1/3 cup water

For mousse:

1/2 cup (4 ounces) fat-free cream cheese at room temperature	1 tablespoon vanilla extract 1 cup macadamia praline 3 large egg whites, at room temperature
1/4 cup (2 ounces) light Neufchâtel cheese at room temperature	1/4 cup granulated sugar 1 cup light whipped topping plus extra for garnish, if desired
1 tablespoon liquid nondairy creamer	

Lightly coat an 8-inch round cake pan with vegetable or canola oil spray and evenly sprinkle in the nuts. To make the praline, in a small saucepan combine the sugar and water. Cook over high heat, undisturbed, until sugar begins to turn light amber in color. As soon as the sugar is getting close to a golden amber, take the pan off the heat and let it continue to caramelize to a deep golden amber, swirling the pan to even out the color. Once the sugar syrup is a deep golden amber, pour it over the nuts. Toss the nuts with a fork to coat them with the caramel. Let the praline cool and harden in the pan.

When the praline is hard, rap the pan on a countertop to break the candy. It will come right out of the pan in large chunks. Place the chunks in a thick plastic bag, or a doubled paper bag, and crush them as fine as you can with a hammer or rolling pin. Transfer praline to food processor fitted with the metal blade and

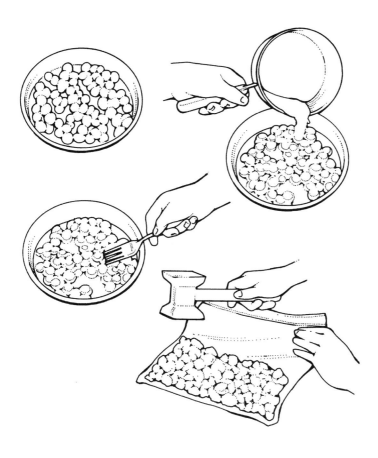

grind in two or three batches until it resembles a coarse meal. Praline will be somewhat sticky due to the oil content of the nuts. Store praline in an airtight container in the refrigerator until ready to use. This keeps the caramel from breaking back down to its liquid form. This recipe makes enough praline for two batches of mousse, and the extra praline will keep in the refrigerator for several months.

To make the mousse, in a food processor fitted with the metal blade, puree cream cheese, Neufchâtel cheese, creamer, and vanilla. Transfer mixture to a large bowl and stir in the 1 cup praline.

In a medium-size mixing bowl that is clean and grease-free, beat the egg whites on medium speed of electric mixer until soft

continued

Custards, Mousses, and Decadent Creations

peaks form. Increase speed to high and sprinkle in the sugar a tablespoon at a time, beating until firm peaks form. Add beaten egg whites and light whipped topping to praline mixture and carefully fold together, using a rubber spatula. You can divide the mousse between 6 individual cups or glasses, or you can chill it as a whole in a large bowl or soufflé dish. Refrigerate for at least 4 hours or overnight before serving.

Serving Suggestions

Try a dollop of light whipped topping sprinkled with some of the extra macadamia praline. It also tastes delicious when drizzled with Chocolate Sauce (page 201). For added texture, top it with Crushed Meringue (page 208).

Variation

You can omit the crushed praline and fold in 2 cups of fresh raspberries for a wonderful raspberry mousse!

Each serving provides

240 Calories   46% Calories from Fat   12 g Fat
29 g Carbohydrates   6 g Protein   82 mg Calcium
0 g Dietary Fiber   186 mg Sodium   11 mg Cholesterol

Tiramisù

12 servings

Yes, it's true! This age-old Italian dessert that has suddenly become all the rage throughout the country has actually found its place among the other lowfat delights in this book. I am very fond of Tiramisù (that's Italian for "pick me up") and did not change it to lowfat proportions carelessly. I knew it had to be good to be worthy of a spot in this book. I have carefully balanced real mascarpone and fat-free cream cheese, along with all of the traditional flavors like sweet Marsala, real vanilla, dark rum, and robust espresso.

Ingredients

- 1 cup espresso or very strong black coffee
- 1 tablespoon granulated sugar
- 2 tablespoons dark rum

- 2 cups (16 ounces) fat-free cream cheese, at room temperature
- 1/3 cup granulated sugar
- 1 tablespoon vanilla extract
- 1 tablespoon dark rum
- 1 tablespoon Marsala wine

- 1 cup (8 ounces) mascarpone cheese

- 1/4 cup (approximately 2 large) egg whites, at room temperature
- 1/3 cup granulated sugar

- approximately 32 ladyfingers (see Special Ingredients)
- 2 tablespoons unsweetened cocoa

continued

You will need an 8-inch square baking pan. In a small bowl combine the coffee, 1 tablespoon sugar, and 2 tablespoons rum. Set aside.

In a large bowl combine cream cheese, 1/3 cup sugar, vanilla, 1 tablespoon rum, and Marsala, and beat on medium speed of electric mixer until smooth and creamy. Mix in the mascarpone on low speed just until it is incorporated.

In a small bowl that is clean and grease-free, beat the egg whites on medium speed of electric mixer until soft peaks form. Increase speed to high and sprinkle in the remaining 1/3 cup sugar, one tablespoon at a time, beating until all of the sugar has been incorporated and mixture has formed firm peaks. Carefully fold beaten egg whites into cheese mixture, using a rubber spatula, just until there are no traces of egg white to be seen.

For final assembly, dip the ladyfingers into the espresso mixture one at a time and line the bottom of the baking dish with them. They need only a 2-second dip into the liquid, otherwise they will absorb too much liquid and become soggy. It should take approximately 16 cookies to line the bottom of the pan, in two rows of eight. Using a rubber spatula, spread half of the cheese mixture

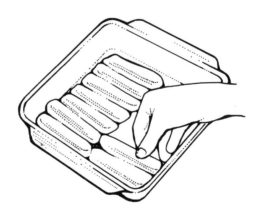

evenly over the first layer of ladyfingers. Now repeat the dipping and layering process with the remaining ladyfingers, laying them carefully on top of the cheese mixture. Spread the other half of the cheese mixture evenly over the second layer of ladyfingers and smooth the top. An icing spatula works well for this.

Refrigerate for at least 6 hours or overnight before serving. To serve, use a fine-mesh sieve to dust the entire surface of Tiramisù with the cocoa. Mark into 12 squares. The easiest way to cut and serve it is to use a small metal spatula that has been dipped in very hot water and wiped dry. This will give a clean cut, and you can easily lift each serving out of the pan.

Serving Suggestions

I definitely like to decorate this dessert with Chocolate Curls (page 191) and then another dusting of cocoa. You may serve it on a pool of Coffee Anglais (page 191), or just decorate it with a few fresh berries. Either way it doesn't need much as it is already a very rich-tasting dessert.

Each serving provides

258 Calories   36% Calories from Fat   9 g Fat
30 g Carbohydrates   8 g Protein   129 mg Calcium
0 g Dietary Fiber   231 mg Sodium   140 mg Cholesterol

Peach Blueberry Cobbler with Cornmeal Crisp

9 servings

The addition of cornmeal makes an exceptionally crisp topping for this delicious cobbler. This dessert is a must when peaches are in season.

For cornmeal crisp:

1/2 cup all-purpose flour
1/4 cup granulated sugar
1/4 cup yellow cornmeal

1/4 cup (1/2 stick) light butter, at room temperature

For filling:

6 medium ripe peaches
3/4 cup blueberries, fresh or frozen
2 teaspoons vanilla extract

1/4 cup firmly packed brown sugar
1/4 cup granulated sugar
1/4 cup cornstarch
1/4 teaspoon salt

To make crisp, combine all crisp ingredients and rub mixture together with your fingers to make coarse crumbs. Set aside while you make the filling.

Preheat oven to 350 degrees F. You will need an 8-inch square baking pan. Cut the peaches in half and remove the pits. Cut each half into 6 segments. Place peaches and blueberries in a large mixing bowl and toss them with the vanilla. In a separate mixing bowl combine both sugars, cornstarch, and salt. Mix well to break up any lumps of brown sugar or cornstarch. Add to the fruit and toss well to coat all of the fruit.

Pour fruit into baking dish, using a spoon or spatula to level out the filling. Top with the cornmeal crisp and bake for approximately 30 to 40 minutes. Crisp should be light golden brown and filling should be bubbly around the edges. Cool for at least 20 minutes before serving. Store tightly wrapped in the refrigerator.

Sweet Deceptions

Serving Suggestions

The obvious choice here would have to be the light whipped topping, second only to a scoop of frozen vanilla yogurt. This cobbler is also very successful when baked individually in large ramekins.

Each serving provides

175 Calories   15% Calories from Fat   3 g Fat
37 g Carbohydrates   2 g Protein   11 mg Calcium
2 g Dietary Fiber   93 mg Sodium   9 mg Cholesterol

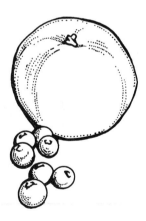

Custards, Mousses, and Decadent Creations

Sierra Mud Slide Pie

12 servings

I named this dessert after watching the news about the California floods in 1995 while I was putting together this book. There were some very big mud slides in the Sierras, so I decided to make something good come out of the whole thing—and the Sierra Mud Slide Pie was born!

For crust:

12 lowfat chocolate Oreo-type cookies, finely crushed	1½ tablespoons light butter, melted

For filling:

1 quart chocolate lowfat frozen yogurt, slightly softened	²/3 cup semisweet chocolate chips
¼ cup liquid nondairy creamer	½ cup (4 ounces) light Neufchâtel cheese, at room temperature
1 tablespoon instant coffee crystals	½ cup marshmallow cream
2 teaspoons vanilla extract	2 tablespoons finely chopped toasted almonds

Lightly coat a 9-inch springform pan with vegetable or canola oil spray. Combine the cookie crumbs and melted butter. Reserve 3 tablespoons of the crumb mixture for sprinkling over the top of the pie, and press the remaining crumb mixture evenly and firmly into the bottom of the pan.

Spread the frozen yogurt over the cookie crust, pressing in a spoonful at a time until all of the crust is covered. It does not have to be perfectly smooth and even. Place in the freezer while preparing filling.

In a small saucepan combine the creamer, coffee crystals, and vanilla. Cook over high heat until it reaches a boil. Remove from heat and add the chocolate chips. Let stand for a couple of minutes before stirring until smooth. If chocolate has not melted completely, you may return it to the stove over medium heat and stir until melted and smooth. Set aside to cool for 10 minutes.

When chocolate mixture has cooled, pour it into a food processor fitted with the metal blade, and add the Neufchâtel cheese. Process until smooth and creamy. Take pan from freezer and dot the entire surface with the marshmallow cream, spreading it out slightly but not completely covering the yogurt. Pour the chocolate mixture over the marshmallow cream, covering the entire surface. Smooth the top with a spatula. Sprinkle surface with the reserved cookie crumbs and the chopped almonds. Cover with plastic wrap and freeze overnight before serving. To unmold, run a hot knife around the edge of the pan and unlatch the side of the pan. When cutting the pie, use the hot-knife method described in General Baking Tips.

Serving Suggestions

This dessert is extremely rich and decadent, so its garnishing should be done with a light hand! Try some light whipped topping, or a drizzle of Gooey Caramel Sauce (page 198).

Each serving provides

228 Calories   42% Calories from Fat   11 g Fat
31 g Carbohydrates   4 g Protein   44 mg Calcium
0 g Dietary Fiber   88 mg Sodium   14 mg Cholesterol

Muffins and Coffee Cakes

Apple Cinnamon Crunch Muffins

Blueberry Muffins

Bran Muffins

Chocolate Chip Muffins

Cherry Cobbler Muffins

Chocolate Cinnamon Muffins

Lemon Poppyseed Muffins

Cinnamon Crunch Muffins

Orange, Almond, and Poppyseed Muffins

Banana Nut Bread

Pumpkin Spice Muffins

Blueberry Frangipane Coffee Cake

Cinnamon Swirl Coffee Cake

Cranberry Bread

Gingerbread Loaves

Frosted Spice Cake

Zucchini Bread

Chapter Six

Muffins and Coffee Cakes

A delicious muffin or a slice of coffee cake is my favorite breakfast, completed of course by a double vanilla latte! I know I'm not alone in this habit. Some of us actually want to have muffins for breakfast, and others make that choice out of necessity—there is no time to sit down to a leisurely breakfast between juggling responsibilities of work, children, and everything in between. Whatever your reasons may be, the fact remains that muffins can be high in fat and calories. I have known of muffins that were as high as 500 calories and 36 grams of fat! Who wants to start their day off that way?

There are some pretty unsavory lowfat muffins out there that have given the term "lowfat" a bad rap. I've tasted plenty of them. Rubbery is the first word that comes to mind. So I did extensive testing of my muffins on some hard-core connoisseurs. I think you'll be just as pleased with the results as they were.

Muffin Success

Creating the perfect muffin can be demanding. You might think, "It's only a muffin, how hard can it possibly be?" As with any baked goodie, muffins require a disciplined hand at following instructions. Make no mistake, no matter how short or easy a recipe looks, you can bet that each one has a specific method to follow to ensure the proper taste and texture. Bottom line: No shortcuts! I have about five years of frustrating shortcut experience on which to base this rule. I know firsthand how easy it is to mess up muffins because I used to consider them easy to make and didn't give them the respect they deserved. The following tips will help answer any questions you might have about how these muffins are made, and ensure that your muffins will be a delicious success!

Pan Preparation

Every muffin recipe in this book will ask you to lightly coat the muffin papers with nonstick cooking spray. Nothing irritates me more than peeling away the paper of my morning muffin only to find that half of my muffin has peeled away with it! This is what will happen if you forget to coat the insides of the muffin papers. This rule doesn't usually apply to regular muffin recipes whose batters have enough butter or oil in them to easily release from the papers. But I have found that these lower-fat muffin batters adhere to the paper like glue. There have been times when I was quite human and forgot to coat the papers, and yet the muffins came loose with great ease. This I cannot explain, so I simply refer to those times as true baking miracles. But I find it better not to play "Muffin Roulette," so to speak—just be sure to coat those muffin papers!

Mixing the Batter

Ask any good baker the secret for successful muffins and he or she is sure to tell you it's all in the way that you handle the batter. Most people tend to overmix the batter, resulting in tough muffins. I have instructed you to mix just until all the ingredients are moist. This means gently stirring or folding the wet ingredients with the dry ingredients until they form a batter which will be rough and lumpy. Many bakers get into trouble at this point because they just can't seem to conquer that urge to work out those lumps into a nice smooth batter. I can hardly blame them because we are used to batters that are smooth and uniform, and it becomes a habit to want them all that way. Muffins are one of the exceptions to the rule, and actually depend on being undermixed for their success. Remember to use either a wooden spoon or, better yet, a trusty old rubber spatula, and fold those ingredients together only to the point where they have combined, and no further. Don't concern yourself with those lumps because they are just part of the magic of muffin-making.

Filling the Muffin Cups

When I make muffins, I want them as big as they can possibly be without having to use a jumbo-size muffin pan. Long gone are the days when you thought you could fill the cups only half or three quarters of the way—at least not with my muffin recipes. Don't hesitate a bit when I ask you to fill them to the rims; this means right up to the tops of the paper muffin cups, or at least very close. I promise they are not going to overflow in the oven. Instead you should get a nice dome top, which is the way a muffin should look as far as I'm concerned. Who wants to eat a measly little flat-topped muffin? I rest my case.

Baking Times and Temperatures

The actual baking is a critical leg of your muffin-making journey. Now that you have so carefully mixed the perfect muffin batter and spooned it clear to the rims into those nicely coated muffin papers, it sure would be a shame to overbake them. Back in General Baking Tips, you read that baking times and temperatures are only guidelines, not unalterable laws. Generally, muffins are baked at a higher temperature than other types of cakes—anywhere from 375 to 400 degrees Fahrenheit. I used to rebel against these high temperatures for fear that my muffins would burn. It took me a while to get over that fear and understand the reasons for doing it that way. I won't be too technical here, but it has to do with the composition of the batter and the fact that you're dealing with a very small amount that doesn't require thirty or forty minutes to bake completely. Therefore it can withstand the higher temperature that causes the batter to rise and bake more quickly, thus creating the domed top of the muffin.

Cooling the Muffins in the Pan

Many people take their muffins out of the oven and immediately dump them out of the pan and onto the counter. I like to cool them in the pan for a little while before removing them. This helps to lock some of the moisture into the muffin that would otherwise escape as steam during the cooling process. For the recipes in this book I have suggested cooling the muffins in the pan for 10 minutes before removing them to cool completely. I chose 10 minutes for the simple fact that most people have only one muffin pan and would be baking all day if they had to wait until the muffins were completely cool before removing them to re-use their pan for another batch of muffins. But if you have the time or the muffin pans you're more than welcome to cool them completely in the pan.

Airtight Containers

When it comes to muffins, I like those rectangular Tupperware-type containers the best because they keep muffins from getting squished. Otherwise those big Ziploc plastic bags work quite well. And last but not least there's the old Saran Wrap over the plate of muffins routine. However, if you know someone who insists on getting their muffins from the grocery store no matter how many wonderful low-fat muffins you send their way, have them give you those nifty little plastic containers that their muffins were packed in. They are easy to wash and can be used over again quite a few times.

Coffee Cakes

You won't find many tips when it comes to coffee cakes. I have kept the methods for mixing coffee cake batters similar to those for mixing muffins so you can refer back to the section on mixing batter for muffins. The baking times and temperatures for the coffee cakes, however, are standard at 350 degrees Fahrenheit and approximate times of 20 to 40 minutes, depending on the particular recipe. Most of the coffee cakes in this book are cooled in the pan and then cut into squares, with the exception of the loaf cakes. As for storage, any of the methods suggested for the muffins are suitable, with the exception of the plastic muffin containers.

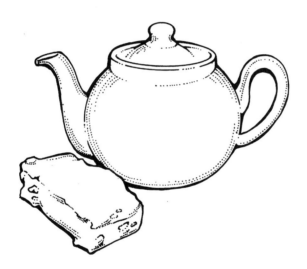

Apple Cinnamon Crunch Muffins

16 muffins

These muffins are especially nice to make in those months when apples seem to be the only fruit in season. They are wonderful on a chilly morning with a cup of coffee or even hot spiced cider!

For streusel topping:

1/3 cup granulated sugar

2 tablespoons all-purpose flour

1 teaspoon ground cinnamon

1 tablespoon light butter, at room temperature

For batter:

1 medium Granny Smith apple

2 1/2 cups all-purpose flour

1 cup granulated sugar

1/2 teaspoon salt

1/2 teaspoon ground allspice

1 tablespoon baking powder

1 teaspoon baking soda

1/2 cup lowfat buttermilk

1/2 cup milk (2 percent)

2 tablespoons canola oil

2 tablespoons light corn syrup

1/3 cup lowfat ricotta cheese

1 large whole egg plus 2 large egg whites

1 tablespoon vanilla extract

Preheat oven to 375 degrees F. Line a muffin pan with paper muffin cups and lightly coat them with vegetable or canola oil spray. To prepare streusel topping, in a small bowl combine sugar, flour, cinnamon, and butter. Rub the mixture together with your fingers to make coarse crumbs, and set aside.

To make batter, remove the core from the apple, quarter it and chop in a food processor until coarse but not pureed. Set apple aside. In a large bowl combine flour, sugar, salt, allspice, baking powder, and baking soda. In a separate bowl combine remaining

Sweet Deceptions

ingredients and whisk until smooth. Stir in the chopped apple and pour mixture into dry ingredients, mixing just until all ingredients are moist. Spoon batter into prepared muffin cups, filling to the rims, and sprinkle the top of each muffin with some of the streusel mixture.

Bake for approximately 20 minutes. Muffins should be light golden brown and a cake tester inserted into the center should come out clean. Cool in pan for 10 minutes before removing to cool completely. Store in an airtight container.

Variation

Apple, Raisin, and Cinnamon Crunch Muffins: Stir $1/2$ cup raisins or sultanas, coarsely chopped, into batter with wet ingredients.

Each serving provides

192 Calories   16% Calories from Fat   3 g Fat
37 g Carbohydrates   4 g Protein   62 mg Calcium
1 g Dietary Fiber   230 mg Sodium   17 mg Cholesterol

(Variation) Each serving provides

194 Calories   15% Calories from Fat   3 g Fat
38 g Carbohydrates   4 g Protein   63 mg Calcium
1 g Dietary Fiber   230 mg Sodium   17 mg Cholesterol

Blueberry Muffins

16 muffins

These are without a doubt the most popular and recognizable muffin around. They are a must to bake when blueberries are in season, as nothing ever tasted as heavenly as a fresh blueberry muffin.

Ingredients

2 1/2 cups all-purpose flour

1 cup granulated sugar

1/2 teaspoon salt

1 tablespoon baking powder

1 teaspoon baking soda

1/2 cup lowfat buttermilk

3/4 cup milk (2 percent)

2 tablespoons canola oil

2 tablespoons light corn syrup

1/3 cup lowfat ricotta cheese

1 large whole egg plus 2 large egg whites

2 teaspoons vanilla extract

1 tablespoon grated lemon peel

1 1/3 cups blueberries, fresh or frozen

Preheat oven to 375 degrees F. Line a muffin pan with paper muffin cups and lightly coat them with vegetable or canola oil spray. In a large mixing bowl combine flour, sugar, salt, baking powder, and baking soda.

In a separate bowl combine all remaining ingredients except for blueberries. Whisk together until smooth. Pour into dry ingredients and mix just until all ingredients are moist. Stir in the blueberries and spoon batter into prepared muffin cups, filling to the rims.

Bake for approximately 20 to 25 minutes. Muffins should be light golden brown and a cake tester inserted into the center should come out clean. Cool in pan for 10 minutes before removing to cool completely. Store in an airtight container.

Sweet Deceptions

Blueberry Streusel Muffins: Combine 1/3 cup granulated sugar, 3 table-spoons flour, and 1 1/2 tablespoons light butter at room temperature. Rub mix-ture together with your fingers to make coarse crumbs. Sprinkle over muffins before baking.

Each serving provides

171 Calories   16% Calories from Fat   3 g Fat
32 g Carbohydrates   4 g Protein   65 mg Calcium
1 g Dietary Fiber   228 mg Sodium   16 mg Cholesterol

(Variation) Each serving provides

196 Calories   16% Calories from Fat   4 g Fat
37 g Carbohydrates   5 g Protein   66 mg Calcium
1 g Dietary Fiber   234 mg Sodium   18 mg Cholesterol

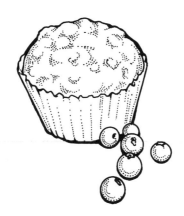

Bran Muffins

14 muffins

I know how boring, dry, and tasteless bran muffins can be. Perhaps that's why no one really gets excited about them. This recipe will change your bran-muffin outlook, as these are rich and robust with the addition of chocolate, coffee, and molasses, and just the right amount of juicy pineapple. Fiber never had it so good!

Ingredients

2 cups all-purpose flour
2 cups wheat bran
1 cup granulated sugar
1 tablespoon unsweetened cocoa
1 tablespoon baking powder
1 teaspoon salt
2/3 cup lowfat buttermilk

1/4 cup black coffee
3/4 cup crushed pineapple, drained
1/3 cup lowfat ricotta cheese
1 tablespoon molasses
2 tablespoons honey
2 large egg whites
1 tablespoon vanilla extract

Preheat oven to 350 degrees F. Line a muffin pan with paper muffin cups and lightly coat them with vegetable or canola oil spray. In a large mixing bowl combine flour, wheat bran, sugar, cocoa, baking powder, and salt.

In a separate mixing bowl combine remaining ingredients and whisk together until smooth. Pour into the dry ingredients and mix just until all ingredients are moist. Spoon batter into prepared muffin cups, filling to the rims.

Bake for 20 to 25 minutes, or until a cake tester inserted into the center comes out with a few moist crumbs. Cool in pan for 10 minutes before removing to cool completely on rack. Store in an airtight container.

Each serving provides

177 Calories   6% Calories from Fat   1 g Fat
40 g Carbohydrates   5 g Protein   68 mg Calcium
4 g Dietary Fiber   247 mg Sodium   3 mg Cholesterol

Sweet Deceptions

Chocolate Chip Muffins

12 muffins

Ingredients

2 1/2 cups all-purpose flour
1 1/4 cups granulated sugar
3/4 teaspoon salt
1 tablespoon baking powder
1 teaspoon baking soda
3 tablespoons mini semi-sweet chocolate chips
1/2 cup lowfat buttermilk

3/4 cup milk (2 percent)
2 tablespoons canola oil
1/3 cup lowfat ricotta cheese
1 large whole egg plus 2 large egg whites
1 tablespoon vanilla extract

Preheat oven to 375 degrees F. Line a muffin pan with paper muffin cups and lightly coat them with vegetable or canola oil spray. In a large bowl combine flour, sugar, salt, baking powder, baking soda, and chocolate chips. In a separate bowl combine remaining ingredients and whisk together until smooth. Pour into dry ingredients and mix just until all the ingredients are moist. Spoon batter into prepared muffin cups, filling to the rims.

Bake for approximately 20 minutes. Muffins should be light golden brown and a cake tester inserted into the center should come out clean. Cool in pan for 10 minutes before removing to cool completely. Store in an airtight container.

Each serving provides

239 Calories   18% Calories from Fat   5 g Fat
43 g Carbohydrates   6 g Protein   86 mg Calcium
1 g Dietary Fiber   342 mg Sodium   21 mg Cholesterol

Cherry Cobbler Muffins

16 muffins

If you love cobbler, these may very well turn out to be your favorite muffins. They are just like eating a miniature cobbler, complete with a fruity filling and a crisp streusel topping. They also make a nice dessert served with a dollop of light whipped topping.

For streusel topping:

3 tablespoons all-purpose flour

1/3 cup granulated sugar

1/4 cup old-fashioned oats

2 tablespoons light butter at room temperature

For batter:

2 1/2 cups all-purpose flour

1 cup granulated sugar

1/2 teaspoon salt

1 tablespoon baking powder

1 teaspoon baking soda

1/2 cup lowfat buttermilk

3/4 cup milk (2 percent)

2 tablespoons canola oil

2 tablespoons light corn syrup

1/3 cup lowfat ricotta cheese

1 large whole egg plus 2 large egg whites

1 tablespoon vanilla extract

1 3/4 cup cherry pie filling

Preheat oven to 375 degrees F. Line a muffin pan with paper muffin cups and lightly coat them with vegetable or canola oil spray. To prepare streusel topping, in a small bowl combine flour, sugar, oats, and butter. Rub the mixture together with your fingers to make coarse crumbs, and set aside.

To prepare batter, in a large bowl combine flour, sugar, salt, baking powder, and baking soda. In a separate bowl combine all remaining ingredients except the cherry filling. Whisk together until smooth and pour into the dry ingredients, mixing just until all ingredients are moist. Spoon batter into prepared muffin cups, fill-

Sweet Deceptions

ing to within a quarter-inch of the rim. Place approximately 1/2 tablespoon of cherry filling in the center of each muffin (for me this worked out to be about 4 cherries per muffin), and then top each muffin with some of the streusel mixture.

Bake for approximately 20 to 25 minutes. Muffins should be light golden brown, and a cake tester inserted just off to the side of the filling should come out clean. Cool in pan for 10 minutes before removing to cool completely. Store in an airtight container.

Each serving provides

230 Calories   15% Calories from Fat   4 g Fat
44 g Carbohydrates   5 g Protein   66 mg Calcium
3 g Dietary Fiber   237 mg Sodium   19 mg Cholesterol

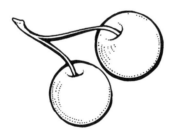

Chocolate Cinnamon Muffins

12 muffins

The pairing up of chocolate and cinnamon makes an unusual but very delicious muffin. Since they are chocolatey, they also make an excellent after-dinner sweet.

Ingredients

2 1/4 cups all-purpose flour
1 1/4 cups granulated sugar
1/2 teaspoon salt
1 tablespoon baking powder
1 teaspoon baking soda
3 tablespoons unsweetened cocoa
1 1/2 teaspoons ground cinnamon

1/2 cup lowfat buttermilk
3/4 cup milk (2 percent)
2 tablespoons canola oil
1/3 cup lowfat ricotta cheese
1 large whole egg plus 2 large egg whites
1 tablespoon vanilla extract

Preheat oven to 375 degrees F. Line a muffin pan with paper muffin cups and lightly coat them with vegetable or canola oil spray. In a large bowl combine flour, sugar, salt, baking powder, baking soda, cocoa, and cinnamon. In a separate bowl combine remaining ingredients and whisk together until smooth. Pour into dry ingredients and mix just until all ingredients are moist. Spoon batter into prepared muffin cups, filling to the rims.

Bake for approximately 20 minutes. Muffins should be light golden brown and a cake tester inserted into the center should come out clean. Cool in pan for 10 minutes before removing to cool completely. Store in an airtight container.

Each serving provides

221 Calories   17% Calories from Fat   4 g Fat
41 g Carbohydrates   6 g Protein   90 mg Calcium
1 g Dietary Fiber   298 mg Sodium   21 mg Cholesterol

Lemon Poppyseed Muffins

14 muffins

These muffins are light and lemony with just the right amount of crunchy poppyseeds and they are perfect in the summertime, especially after a light lunch or with afternoon tea.

Ingredients

2 1/2 cups all-purpose flour
1 cup granulated sugar
1/2 teaspoon salt
1 tablespoon baking powder
1 1/2 tablespoons poppy seeds
1/2 cup lowfat buttermilk
1/2 cup milk (2 percent)
1/4 cup fresh lemon juice

2 tablespoons canola oil
1/3 cup lowfat ricotta cheese
1 large whole egg plus 2 large egg whites
1/2 teaspoon vanilla extract
2 tablespoons grated lemon peel

Preheat oven to 375 degrees F. Line a muffin pan with paper muffin cups and lightly coat them with vegetable or canola oil spray. In a large bowl combine flour, sugar, salt, baking powder, and poppy seeds. In a separate bowl combine remaining ingredients and whisk together until smooth. Pour into dry ingredients and mix just until all ingredients are moist. Spoon batter into prepared muffin cups, filling to the rims.

Bake for approximately 20 minutes. Muffins should be light golden brown and a cake tester inserted into the center should come out clean. Cool in pan for 10 minutes before removing to cool completely. Store in an airtight container.

Each serving provides

183 Calories   18% Calories from Fat   4 g Fat
33 g Carbohydrates   5 g Protein   84 mg Calcium
1 g Dietary Fiber   176 mg Sodium   18 mg Cholesterol

Cinnamon Crunch Muffins

12 muffins

These are as simple and elegant as a muffin can get. They are moist and plain with a crunchy cinnamon streusel topping, and are excellent when paired up with a flavored coffee such as hazelnut or vanilla.

For streusel topping:

1/3 cup granulated sugar
2 tablespoons all-purpose flour
1 teaspoon ground cinnamon

1 tablespoon light butter, at room temperature

For batter:

2 1/2 cups all-purpose flour
1 cup granulated sugar
1/2 teaspoon salt
1 tablespoon baking powder
1 teaspoon baking soda
1/4 teaspoon ground cinnamon
1/2 cup lowfat buttermilk

3/4 cup milk (2 percent)
2 tablespoons canola oil
2 tablespoons light corn syrup
1/3 cup lowfat ricotta cheese
1 large whole egg plus 2 large egg whites
1 tablespoon vanilla extract

Preheat oven to 375 degrees F. Line a muffin pan with paper muffin cups and lightly coat them with vegetable or canola oil spray. To prepare streusel topping, in a small bowl combine sugar, flour, cinnamon, and butter. Rub mixture together with your fingers to make coarse crumbs, and set aside.

To prepare batter, in a large bowl combine flour, sugar, salt, baking powder, baking soda, and cinnamon. In a separate bowl combine remaining ingredients and whisk together until smooth. Pour into dry ingredients and mix just until all ingredients are moist. Spoon batter into prepared muffin cups, filling to the rims, and top each muffin with some of the streusel mixture.

Bake for approximately 20 minutes. Muffins should be light golden brown and a cake tester inserted into the center should come out clean. Cool in the pan for 10 minutes before removing to cool completely. Store in an airtight container.

Each serving provides

249 Calories   16% Calories from Fat   4 g Fat
47 g Carbohydrates   6 g Protein   86 mg Calcium
1 g Dietary Fiber   308 mg Sodium   23 mg Cholesterol

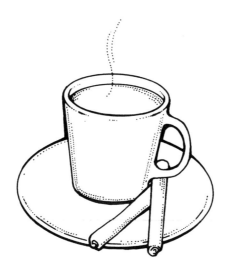

Orange, Almond, and Poppyseed Muffins

14 muffins

Ingredients

2 1/2 cups all-purpose flour	1/3 cup lowfat ricotta cheese
1 cup granulated sugar	1 large whole egg plus 2 large egg whites
1/2 teaspoon salt	
1 tablespoon baking powder	2 teaspoons vanilla extract
2 1/2 tablespoons poppy seeds	1 1/2 teaspoons almond extract
1/2 cup lowfat buttermilk	
1/4 cup milk (2 percent)	1 tablespoon grated orange peel
1/2 cup orange juice	
2 tablespoons canola oil	

Preheat oven to 375 degrees F. Line a muffin pan with paper muffin cups and lightly coat them with vegetable or canola oil spray. In a large bowl combine flour, sugar, salt, baking powder, and poppy seeds. In a separate bowl combine remaining ingredients and whisk together until smooth. Spoon batter into prepared muffin cups, filling to the rims.

Bake for approximately 20 minutes. Muffins should be light golden brown and a cake tester inserted into the center should come out clean. Cool in the pan for 10 minutes before removing to cool completely. Store in an airtight container.

Each serving provides

189 Calories   18% Calories from Fat   4 g Fat
34 g Carbohydrates   5 g Protein   87 mg Calcium
1 g Dietary Fiber   174 mg Sodium   18 mg Cholesterol

Banana Nut Bread

20 servings

Ingredients

2 1/2 cups all-purpose flour
1/2 cup granulated sugar
1/2 cup firmly packed
    brown sugar
1 teaspoon salt
1 tablespoon baking
    powder
1 teaspoon baking soda
1 teaspoon ground
    allspice
1 teaspoon ground
    cinnamon

1/2 cup (1 1/2 ounces)
    ground pecans
1/3 cup lowfat buttermilk
1 1/2 medium bananas, ripe
1/3 cup milk (2 percent)
1/3 cup lowfat ricotta
    cheese
2 tablespoons honey
2 large egg whites
2 tablespoons canola oil
1 tablespoon vanilla
    extract

Preheat oven to 350 degrees F. Lightly coat two 8 × 3 3/4-inch loaf pans with vegetable or canola oil spray. In a large bowl combine flour, both sugars, salt, baking powder, baking soda, spices, and ground pecans.

In a food processor fitted with the metal blade puree the buttermilk and bananas until smooth. In another bowl combine remaining ingredients. Add the banana puree and whisk together until smooth. Pour into dry ingredients and mix just until all ingredients are moist.

Divide batter between the two loaf pans and bake for approximately 35 to 40 minutes or until a cake tester inserted into the center comes out clean. Remove from the pans and cool completely on a rack. Store in an airtight container.

Each serving provides

157 Calories   21% Calories from Fat   4 g Fat
28 g Carbohydrates   3 g Protein   54 mg Calcium
1 g Dietary Fiber   231 mg Sodium   2 mg Cholesterol

Pumpkin Spice Muffins

12 muffins

Without a doubt, these are the muffins to be making during the holidays. However, I wrote this book during the spring and summer months and they tasted every bit as good. I almost forgot what season it was, as I felt like going Christmas shopping!

Ingredients

2¹/₂ cups all-purpose flour
¹/₂ cup granulated sugar
¹/₂ cup firmly packed brown sugar
¹/₂ teaspoon salt
1 tablespoon baking powder
1 teaspoon baking soda
1 teaspoon ground nutmeg
1 teaspoon ground cinnamon
1 teaspoon ground ginger

¹/₃ cup lowfat buttermilk
¹/₂ cup milk (2 percent)
2 tablespoons canola oil
¹/₃ cup lowfat ricotta cheese
1 large whole egg plus 1 large egg white
1 tablespoon vanilla extract
¹/₂ cup plus 2 tablespoons (5 ounces) canned pumpkin

Preheat oven to 375 degrees F. Line a muffin pan with paper muffin cups and lightly coat them with vegetable or canola oil spray. In a large bowl combine flour, both sugars, salt, baking powder, baking soda, and spices. In a separate bowl combine remaining ingredients and whisk together until smooth. Pour into dry ingredients and mix just until all ingredients are moist. Spoon batter into prepared muffin cups, filling to the rims.

Bake for approximately 20 minutes. Muffins should be light golden brown and a cake tester inserted into the center should come out clean. Cool in pan for 10 minutes before removing to cool completely. Store in an airtight container.

Each serving provides

223 Calories   16% Calories from Fat   4 g Fat
41 g Carbohydrates   5 g Protein   94 mg Calcium
1 g Dietary Fiber   293 mg Sodium   21 mg Cholesterol

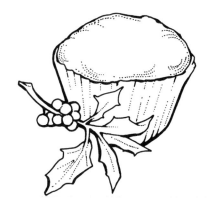

Blueberry Frangipane Coffee Cake

12 squares

Blueberry coffee cake is certainly delicious all on its own, but almond extract and almond streusel add a different and unique taste to an old favorite.

For streusel topping:

2 tablespoons pure almond paste

2 tablespoons light butter, at room temperature

1/4 cup firmly packed brown sugar

1/4 cup plus 2 tablespoons all-purpose flour

For batter:

2 cups all-purpose flour

3/4 cup granulated sugar

3/4 teaspoon salt

1 tablespoon baking powder

1/2 cup lowfat buttermilk

1/2 cup milk (2 percent)

1/3 cup lowfat ricotta cheese

2 large egg whites

1 tablespoon vanilla extract

2 tablespoons canola oil

1/2 teaspoon almond extract

1 cup blueberries, fresh or frozen

Preheat oven to 350 degrees F. Lightly coat an 8-inch square baking pan with vegetable or canola oil spray. To prepare streusel topping, combine almond paste, butter, brown sugar, and flour. Rub mixture together with your fingers to make coarse crumbs. Set aside.

To prepare batter, in a large bowl combine flour, sugar, salt, and baking powder. In a separate bowl combine remaining ingredients except blueberries. Whisk together until smooth. Pour into dry ingredients and mix just until all ingredients are moist. Pour into prepared pan and sprinkle the blueberries evenly over the surface of the batter. Sprinkle the streusel topping evenly over the blueberries.

Bake for 35 to 40 minutes or until a cake tester inserted into the center comes out clean. Cool completely in pan on a rack before cutting. Store in an airtight container.

Each serving provides

227 Calories 20% Calories from Fat 5 g Fat
40 g Carbohydrates 5 g Protein 87 mg Calcium
1 g Dietary Fiber 259 mg Sodium 7 mg Cholesterol

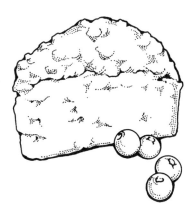

Cinnamon Swirl Coffee Cake

12 squares

For cinnamon swirl:

1/4 cup firmly packed
brown sugar

1/3 cup granulated sugar

1 tablespoon ground
cinnamon

1/4 teaspoon salt

2 tablespoons light butter,
melted

2 tablespoons light corn
syrup

For batter:

2 1/2 cups all-purpose flour

1 cup granulated sugar

1/2 teaspoon salt

1 tablespoon baking
powder

1/2 cup lowfat buttermilk

3/4 cup nondairy liquid
creamer

1/3 cup lowfat ricotta
cheese

1 large whole egg plus
2 large egg whites

2 tablespoons canola oil

1 tablespoon vanilla
extract

Preheat oven to 350 degrees F. Lightly coat a 9 × 13-inch baking pan with vegetable or canola oil spray. To prepare cinnamon swirl, combine brown sugar, granulated sugar, cinnamon, and salt. Stir in melted butter and corn syrup until smooth, and set aside.

To prepare batter, in a large bowl combine flour, sugar, salt, and baking powder. In a separate bowl combine remaining ingredients and whisk together until smooth. Pour into the dry ingredients and mix just until all ingredients are moist. Pour batter into prepared pan and dot the entire surface with the cinnamon swirl mixture. Using a knife or icing spatula, marble the cinnamon mixture into the batter by swirling it around. Do not overmix so that the design will remain after it is baked.

Bake for 25 to 30 minutes or until a cake tester inserted into the center comes out clean. Cool completely in the pan on a rack. Store in an airtight container.

Each serving provides

280 Calories   19% Calories from Fat   6 g Fat
51 g Carbohydrates   5 g Protein   79 mg Calcium
1 g Dietary Fiber   270 mg Sodium   24 mg Cholesterol

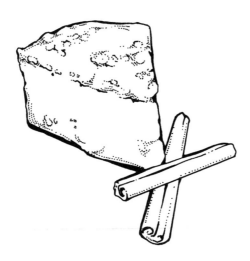

Cranberry Bread

20 servings

I love cranberries, but unfortunately they are a seasonal fruit and I can never seem to remember to stock up when they are around. I know I'm not the only one with this problem, so I came up with this recipe which is made with canned whole cranberry sauce. It actually turns out a delicious bread for those times when you just have to have something cranberry.

Ingredients

2 1/2 cups all-purpose flour
3/4 cup granulated sugar
2 teaspoons baking powder
1/2 teaspoon baking soda
1/2 teaspoon salt
1 teaspoon ground ginger
1/3 cup lowfat buttermilk
1/4 cup orange juice
1/4 cup lowfat ricotta cheese
3 tablespoons canola oil
2 large egg whites
1 tablespoon vanilla extract
1 can (16 ounces) whole berry cranberry sauce

Preheat oven to 350 degrees F. Lightly coat two 8 × 3 3/4-inch loaf pans with vegetable or canola oil spray. In a large bowl combine flour, sugar, baking powder, baking soda, salt, and ground ginger. In a separate bowl combine remaining ingredients except cranberry sauce. Whisk together until smooth. Whisk in the cranberry sauce. Pour into the dry ingredients and mix just until all ingredients are moist.

Pour batter into prepared pans and bake for 35 to 45 minutes or until a cake tester inserted into the center comes out with a few moist crumbs on it. Cool in pans on a rack for 10 minutes before turning out onto a rack to cool completely. Store in an airtight container.

Each serving provides

159 Calories 15% Calories from Fat 3 g Fat
31 g Carbohydrates 3 g Protein 31 mg Calcium
1 g Dietary Fiber 141 mg Sodium 1 mg Cholesterol

Gingerbread Loaves

20 servings

I happen to love the taste of gingerbread in any form, from cookies to cake to fancy houses! Thus my inspiration for this recipe, which happens to be delicious for breakfast.

Ingredients

2 1/2 cups all-purpose flour
1/2 cup granulated sugar
1/2 cup brown sugar
1 tablespoon baking powder
1 teaspoon baking soda
1 teaspoon salt
1 tablespoon ground ginger
1 teaspoon ground allspice

1/2 cup lowfat buttermilk
2/3 cup milk (2 percent)
1/3 cup lowfat ricotta cheese
1/4 cup molasses
2 tablespoons canola oil
2 large egg whites
1 tablespoon vanilla extract

Preheat oven to 350 degrees F. Lightly coat two 8 × 3 3/4-inch loaf pans with vegetable or canola oil spray. In a large bowl combine flour, both sugars, baking powder, baking soda, salt, and spices. In a separate bowl combine remaining ingredients and whisk together until smooth. Pour into the dry ingredients and mix just until all ingredients are moist.

Pour into prepared loaf pans and bake for 30 to 40 minutes or until a cake tester inserted into the center comes out clean. Cool in pans on a rack for 10 minutes before turning out onto a rack to cool completely. Store in an airtight container.

Each serving provides

140 Calories   14% Calories from Fat   2 g Fat
27 g Carbohydrates   3 g Protein   61 mg Calcium
1 g Dietary Fiber   239 mg Sodium   3 mg Cholesterol

Frosted Spice Cake

12 squares

This coffee cake has such a homey, comforting flavor, you'll want it for more than just breakfast. It also makes a nice, quick dessert when you don't have much time for baking.

For cake:

2 cups all-purpose flour	1/2 cup lowfat buttermilk
1 cup granulated sugar	1/3 cup milk (2 percent)
3/4 teaspoon salt	2 tablespoons canola oil
2 1/2 teaspoons baking powder	2 tablespoons light corn syrup
1/4 teaspoon baking soda	1/4 cup lowfat ricotta cheese
1 teaspoon ground allspice	1 large whole egg plus 2 large egg whites
1 teaspoon ground cinnamon	1 tablespoon vanilla extract
1 teaspoon ground ginger	
1/2 teaspoon ground cloves	

For icing:

1/2 cup powdered sugar	1 tablespoon orange juice

Preheat oven to 350 degrees F. Lightly coat an 8-inch square baking pan with vegetable or canola oil spray. In a large bowl combine flour, sugar, salt, baking powder, baking soda, and spices. In a separate bowl combine remaining batter ingredients and whisk together until smooth. Pour into dry ingredients and mix just until all ingredients are moist.

Pour into prepared pan and bake for 20 to 30 minutes or until a cake tester inserted into the center comes out clean. Cool completely in pan on a rack before icing cake.

To prepare icing, in a small bowl combine powdered sugar and orange juice, and stir to make a smooth icing. Spread over cooled cake and let icing set for 30 minutes before cutting. Store in an airtight container.

Each serving provides

214 Calories   15% Calories from Fat   4 g Fat
41 g Carbohydrates   5 g Protein   68 mg Calcium
1 g Dietary Fiber   261 mg Sodium   20 mg Cholesterol

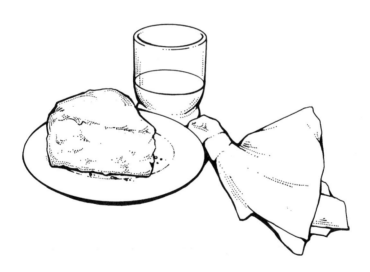

Zucchini Bread

20 servings

Ingredients

2¹/₂ cups all-purpose flour
¹/₂ cup granulated sugar
¹/₂ cup firmly packed brown sugar
1 teaspoon salt
1 tablespoon baking powder
1 teaspoon baking soda
1 teaspoon ground allspice
1 teaspoon ground cinnamon

¹/₃ cup lowfat buttermilk
¹/₂ cup milk (2 percent)
¹/₃ cup lowfat ricotta cheese
2 tablespoons honey
1 large whole egg plus 1 large egg white
1 tablespoon vanilla extract
¹/₄ cup canola oil
1¹/₄ cups grated zucchini

Preheat oven to 350 degrees F. Lightly coat two 8 × 3³/₄-inch loaf pans with vegetable or canola oil spray. In a large bowl combine flour, both sugars, salt, baking powder, baking soda, and spices. In a separate bowl combine remaining ingredients except the zucchini. Whisk together until smooth and stir in the grated zucchini. Add to dry ingredients and mix just until all ingredients are moist.

Pour into prepared pans and bake for 35 to 40 minutes or until a cake tester inserted into the center comes out clean. Remove loaves from pans and cool completely on a rack. Store in an airtight container.

Each serving provides

151 Calories   22% Calories from Fat   4 g Fat
26 g Carbohydrates   3 g Protein   58 mg Calcium
1 g Dietary Fiber   233 mg Sodium   13 mg Cholesterol

Finishing Touches

Light Whipped Topping

A la Mode

Chocolate Decor

The Quintessential Chocolate Curl

Little Froufrous

Crème Anglaise

Gooey Caramel Sauce

Gem Caramel Sauce

Chocolate Sauce

Raspberry Sauce

Strawberry Sauce

Orange Sauce

Apricot Puree

Chocolate Ganache

Chocolate Icing

Crushed Meringue

Chapter Seven

---

finishing Touches

Although I went to great lengths to make the desserts in this book look and taste as decadent as the real things, there are a number of ways to serve and garnish them, and in some cases make them even more decadent. This chapter has been devised especially for this purpose. Here are some great ideas, whether you're making something special for your family, or throwing a dinner party and want the desserts to look as fancy as the ones you've enjoyed at your favorite restaurant.

On the following pages you'll find everything from recipes for dessert sauces—from caramel and chocolate to fresh fruit purees—right down to any garnish imaginable, from simple fresh berries and fresh mint to dark chocolate curls and toasted nuts. Along with the recipes and suggested techniques, I have also provided the nutritional breakdown for the more decadent garnishes in case you would like to know just how many extra calories and fat grams you are adding to the dessert.

Light Whipped Topping

Why do some desserts seem incomplete without a dollop of whipped cream perched on top? Is it so hard to resist the temptation of real heavy cream whipped to dreamy soft peaks with just the right amount of sugar and vanilla? I don't know about you, but I get weak in the knees just thinking about it. Luckily, I remember my backside, and my common sense intervenes just in time with a loud and clear

"I don't think so!" Now I'm not saying that you have to swear off the real stuff forever. Just lower your standards a bit and learn to settle for a light whipped topping. You're already getting a decadent lowfat dessert; even some of those are calling out for that final touch of something creamy and whipped. Don't think for a second that it's okay to have real whipped cream just because your dessert is less sinful—that train of thought will get you nothing but trouble! I'm a chef, and one of the worst critics when it comes to real and artificial, but I also try to live in a world of reality. I am writing all of this, obviously, for those of you who swear by the real thing and wouldn't dream of using anything else. I want you to know that Cool Whip Light really does the job when you're looking for that "mouth feel" that you get from real whipped cream. Take it or leave it, this is my solution to that particular dilemma. It sure worked when I was indulging in a piece of Caramel Pecan and Coconut Tart!

A la Mode

Good old ice cream, real, heavy, rich cream lurking behind an irresistible frozen form—don't go reaching for that Ben and Jerry's! Remember, self control. Also remember that lowfat frozen yogurt isn't what it used to be, and that there are some pretty decent brands out there to choose from if you're looking for something to fill the ice cream void effectively. Read the nutritional information on the package to be sure of what you're getting.

Chocolate Decor

I love to accent desserts with chocolate decorations of all shapes and sizes. You can buy many kinds, such as chocolate twigs, shells, leaves, and nonpareils. Check the package for calories and fat grams per serving and add them to your dessert totals.

The most popular decoration has to be the classic chocolate curl; it will never go out of style. Just because this is a lowfat dessert book doesn't mean you can't shower your tortes with them every now and then. Just do it with a discreet hand and lots of self control!

I cannot be exact on how many calories and fat grams are in each chocolate curl, but if you're only using a few on each dessert, why worry about it? However, if you plan to pile them high on a cake like Death by Chocolate or White Chocolate Raspberry Revel, here is a very close estimation for a larger amount of chocolate curls, followed by some tips for making great curls.

I started with an 8-ounce bar of semisweet chocolate that was 6 inches long by 3 1/2 inches wide by 1 inch thick and curled off about half of it, which gave me approximately 4 ounces of chocolate in curled form. Those 4 ounces of chocolate curls have approximately 600 calories and 40 grams of fat as a whole. Keep in mind, that's a lot of chocolate curls, and once you divide them up, the numbers are reduced quite a bit. 20 servings = 30 calories and 2 grams of fat per serving. 16 servings = 37.5 calories and 2.5 grams of fat per serving. And 12 servings = 50 calories and 3.33 grams of fat per serving. These numbers aren't always going to be exact, and they will change when dealing with white or milk chocolate, but they are close enough for you to get an idea of how many extra calories and fat grams you are adding on. Just use the above formula.

The Quintessential Chocolate Curl

They're so easy to make if you remember the little tricks, and are patient with the chocolate. If it's a hot, sticky day, don't even bother—the curls will never happen!

#1. Always use a fresh bar of chocolate that is still in temper. "Temper" refers to the crystallized state of the chocolate. If chocolate is in temper, it will be smooth and uniform in color all the way through. The chocolate should have no sign of bloom (white streaks and blotches); this happens when the chocolate has been stored at too high a temperature. Seventy degrees and higher will cause some of the fat crystals in the chocolate to melt and rise to the surface; this is what causes the bloom.

Bringing chocolate to a tempered state requires a strict method of melting and cooling to specific temperatures. This process is what makes the chocolate so even and smooth in appearance and texture. Once tempered chocolate has been melted down, it is then considered out of temper. If it is allowed to cool without going through the tempering process, it will look dull with white patches (bloom) and the texture will be grainy rather than smooth. This is why I always use tempered chocolate to make my curls, and unless they are on a torte that must be refrigerated, I store any extra chocolate curls in an airtight container at room temperature, provided that room temperature doesn't exceed 75 degrees Fahrenheit. I have found that the chocolate will not develop serious bloom between 70 and 75 degrees. In fact, at these temperatures the chocolate is just right for making curls. However, keep in mind, when talking about chocolate there are always going to be exceptions depending on the type and quality of the chocolate. This concludes my chocolate lecture, but if you'd like a more in-depth explanation on this topic I highly recommend reading the book *Chocolate Artistry* by Elaine Gonzalez.

#2. Tools of the trade are everything. I have seen chocolate curled and shaved in every way possible, but to me, the easiest tool to use is a plain old metal potato peeler. You may have to try out more than one because I have found that the angle of the blades differs slightly from peeler to peeler, and that can affect the way the chocolate curls.

#3. As I mentioned earlier, temperature is very important. For curls, the chocolate cannot be too cold or too warm. I find that if the chocolate is between 70 and 75 degrees Fahrenheit, the best curls can be achieved. You can tell if the temperature is right just by touching it. It shouldn't be so warm that you can press on it and leave an imprint. The best test of all is to run the peeler across it and see what happens!

#4. Always work with a piece of chocolate big enough for you to hold onto without too much trouble. This makes for better curls. The longer the bar of chocolate, the greater the surface to curl, making for some really nice curlicued chocolate!—and fewer peeled fingers, if you get my drift.

#5. It's all in the wrist. The best way to get comfortable at making chocolate curls is to practice different techniques. I always begin with a large rectangle of chocolate and hold it from the bottom, with the edge facing up. Run the peeler across the top edge just like peeling a carrot. You may have to experiment a bit to find the right angle to make the chocolate curl. Be sure to rotate the chocolate in order to curl off all the sides. The warmth from your hands will help keep the chocolate soft enough to curl. Remember to curl onto a large plate or cookie sheet, and let the curls cool and set a bit before placing them on a cake or torte. You can put them in the refrigerator for a couple of minutes to harden before using them, allowing you to handle them with less breakage. I find the best way to handle chocolate curls is with a metal icing spatula. It allows you to pick them up without touching them, as they are very fragile, and place them on top of a cake or other dessert with great ease.

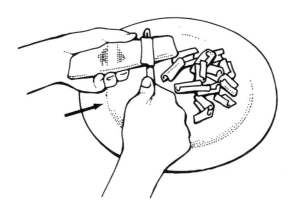

Little Froufrous

Here are some simple things you can add to a dessert to make its presentation more special. Sometimes it's the simple things that seem to add the most to a dessert.

Cocoa and Powdered Sugar

These are very simple ways to dress up the simplest cakes, making them look so elegant! Use a fine-mesh sieve to cover the entire surface of a plain cake with a delicate dusting of unsweetened cocoa or powdered sugar, depending on the type of cake. If you would like a design, lay a paper doily on top of the cake and then dust with a contrasting color. Carefully lift the doily off to reveal a beautiful pattern stenciled onto the surface of the cake. The most dramatic presentation is to top a cake or dessert with chocolate curls and then sift cocoa or powdered sugar over them, cocoa over white chocolate curls and powdered sugar over dark chocolate curls. These are very stunning effects on a cake and you're sure to get a lot of ooohs and aaaahhhs! One tablespoon of unsweetened cocoa has 60 calories and 1.5 grams of fat. One tablespoon of powdered sugar has 30 calories and 0 fat.

Fresh Mint

I can't even imagine a piece of dessert on a plate without a vibrant green sprig of fresh mint. Virtually calorie-free, it is one of the most popular ways to garnish a dessert, and it's edible as well! There are many different types of mint to choose from, each one having its own fragrance and appearance. The old standbys are peppermint and spearmint, but I have also used English mint and pineapple mint as well. Be sure to experiment with them, and taste them as well. You can decorate with whole sprigs, single leaves, or even julienne a few leaves and sprinkle them around or on top of the dessert. Regardless of whatever other garnish or finishing touch you use, you can always add mint as well—I do.

Fresh Fruit and Berries

Nothing looks prettier on a dessert plate than fresh berries—when they are in season, of course. They add color, texture, and dimension without adding many calories. A few fresh berries added to a plate will only add on about 6 or 8 calories for raspberries, blackberries, blueberries, and the like. Strawberries will add about 12 to 15 calories. Try combining different berries for a colorful effect. You can also make strawberry fans by making 4 slices into the berry starting from the bottom, cutting towards the stem, but stopping just short of it. Then separate the slices by fanning them out.

Aside from berries, you can choose a number of different fruits for only a few calories per serving. I have used everything from sliced or wedged kiwi fruit and orange segments, to mangos and papayas cut into delicate, paper-thin slices. Use your imagination as well as whatever your heart desires for added colors and flavors.

Edible Flowers

These make a very elegant garnish when it comes to desserts. The most commonly used are pansies, violets, rose petals, and Johnny jump-ups. There are other interesting choices such as nasturtiums, marigolds, and chrysanthemums. Just ask anyone who deals in edible flowers, and be sure to buy them from a reputable dealer such as a gourmet food store or a local herb farm. Also make sure they are pesticide-free. Do not attempt to garnish your desserts with just any kind of flower because many of them are not edible and can be very toxic.

Toasted Nuts

This is a fun way to garnish any of those chocolate or caramel creations, especially if you have decided to sauce the plate with custard, caramel, or chocolate sauce. You can use nuts whole, roughly chopped, or finely ground, depending on the look you want. I most often use almonds, pecans, hazelnuts, and pistachios for their beautiful green color. You can sprinkle one or many kinds of ground nuts on a sauced plate, or you can leave them whole and strategically place them around or on the dessert. I have provided a list of different types of nuts and their calories and fat content for an $1/8$-ounce serving of whole nuts. I can't be exact, but I approximate about 5 nuts per portion, and a few more when it comes to the peanuts and pistachios because they are smaller.

	Calories	Fat grams
Almonds	20.00	1.87
Brazil nuts	3.12	2.37
Cashews	20.62	1.62
Hazelnuts	22.5	2.25
Macadamia nuts	25.62	2.75
Peanuts	20.5	1.73
Pecans	23.75	2.37
Pistachios	20.62	1.75
Walnuts, quartered	21.87	2.12

Crème Anglaise (Vanilla Custard Sauce)

8 servings
Serving size: 3 tablespoons

Crème Anglaise is the ultimate dessert sauce, not only because its satiny texture is the perfect substitute for dollops of whipped cream or scoops of ice cream, but because when you ladle a pool of it onto a dessert plate, it creates the perfect canvas on which to splash other sauces and garnishes. You can be simple or extravagant, depending on the occasion.

Ingredients

2 large egg yolks
1/4 cup granulated sugar
1 1/2 teaspoons cornstarch
1/2 cup liquid nondairy creamer

1 cup milk (2 percent)
1 tablespoon vanilla extract

In a small saucepan combine the egg yolks and sugar and whisk together until creamy. Add the cornstarch, creamer, milk, and vanilla and whisk together until combined and cornstarch has dissolved. Cook over medium-high heat, stirring constantly with a wooden spoon to prevent any scorching on the bottom of the pan. Continue to cook until mixture thickens and coats the back of the spoon. Remove from heat and transfer to another container to cool. The best way to cool a custard sauce is to place it over a bowl of ice water and stir it until the temperature comes down to room temperature, then cover it and store in the refrigerator. This will prevent a skin from forming on the top of the custard as it cools.

Variation

Coffee Anglaise: Add 1 tablespoon of instant coffee crystals to mixture before cooking and stir to dissolve.

Cocoa Anglaise: Whisk 2 tablespoons sifted unsweetened cocoa into the finished custard sauce.

Each serving provides

78 Calories   35% Calories from Fat   3 g Fat
9 g Carbohydrates   2 g Protein   44 mg Calcium
0 g Dietary Fiber   24 mg Sodium   56 mg Cholesterol

Gooey Caramel Sauce

12 servings
Serving size: 2 tablespoons

If you thought lowfat desserts meant giving up gooey, stretchy caramel sauce, guess again. I know that nothing says sin like true caramel, loaded down with real heavy cream and great gobs of sweet butter. Through some serious experimentation, I managed to come up with a very worthy substitute. You'll find it a little bit lighter than true caramel sauce, but every bit as decadent, gooey, and caramel-like as the real thing.

Ingredients

½   cup liquid nondairy creamer

½   cup sweetened lowfat condensed milk

1½ cups granulated sugar

½   cup water

1   teaspoon salt

2   teaspoons vanilla extract

2   teaspoons butter-flavored extract

Whisk together the creamer and condensed milk and set aside. In a medium-size saucepan combine the sugar, water, and salt. Cook over high heat, undisturbed, until sugar begins to turn light amber in color. As soon as the sugar is getting close to a golden amber take the pan off the heat and let it continue to caramelize to a deep golden amber, swirling the pan to even out the color. Once the sugar is a deep golden amber, carefully pour in the creamer mixture. It will bubble and steam at first. Use a whisk to stir the mixture to dissolve the caramel into the cream; the caramel should be smooth and free of any lumps of undissolved sugar. Whisk in the vanilla and butter flavor. Cool to room temperature before transferring to an airtight container and storing in the refrigerator. This sauce will keep for 1 month in the refrigerator and can be served warm. Reheat in the microwave or warm in a small saucepan over medium-low heat.

Each serving provides

144 Calories   5% Calories from Fat   1 g Fat
33 g Carbohydrates   1 g Protein   34 mg Calcium
0 g Dietary Fiber   196 mg Sodium   0 mg Cholesterol

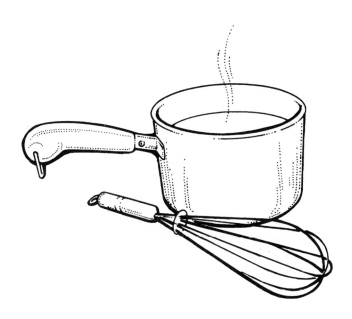

Finishing Touches

Gem Caramel Sauce

6 servings
Serving size: 2 tablespoons

This is caramel in its purest form, before the addition of the cream and butter that transform it into the gooey, stretchy mass that we can never seem to get enough of. This sauce has a very elegant and light taste, and is very similar in texture to honey or corn syrup. Since no ingredients other than water are added to the sugar once it has caramelized, it remains clear, and reminds me of a pool of topaz or amber. Perhaps that's why I named it Gem Caramel. It is very beautiful when pooled under a dessert, or splashed across a pool of custard sauce.

Ingredients

1 cup granulated sugar
1/4 cup water

1/3 to 1/2 cup very hot water

In a small saucepan combine the sugar and 1/4 cup water. Cook over high heat, undisturbed, until sugar begins to turn light amber in color. As soon as the sugar is getting close to a golden amber, take the pan off the heat and let it continue to caramelize to a deep golden amber, swirling the pan to even out the color. Once the sugar is a deep golden amber, carefully pour in the hot water. The caramel will spatter and steam, so be sure to stand back until it settles down. I have found the easiest and safest way to add the hot water is with a turkey baster because it keeps your hand at a reasonable distance from the spattering caramel. When the caramel does settle down, stir it with a whisk to make sure all of the caramelized sugar dissolves into the water, making a smooth liquid. Cool in the pan to room temperature. As the caramel cools, it will thicken. Transfer to an airtight container and store in the refrigerator. If the sauce gets too thick you can thin it out with a little bit of water.

Each serving provides

120 Calories   0% Calories from Fat   0 g Fat
32 g Carbohydrates   0 g Protein   0 mg Calcium
0 g Dietary Fiber   1 mg Sodium   0 mg Cholesterol

Chocolate Sauce

10 servings
Serving size: 2 tablespoons

This is a satiny chocolate sauce that will have no problem holding its own when paired up with such desserts as Death by Chocolate and Chocolate Raspberry Sanctuary. It also works well when transferred to a squeeze bottle and splashed across other sauces.

Ingredients

1/3 cup liquid nondairy creamer

1/4 cup dark corn syrup

1 cup semisweet chocolate chips

In a small saucepan, combine creamer and corn syrup, and place over medium-high heat until mixture reaches a boil. Remove from heat and add the chocolate chips. Stir until smooth. If chocolate does not melt completely you can return it to the stove over medium heat and continue to stir until it is completely melted and smooth. Remove from heat and cool completely before storing in an airtight container in the refrigerator. To use, simply warm the sauce in the microwave on medium-high for a few seconds at a time until the sauce is of the right consistency to pour. You can also warm it on the stove over very low heat.

Each serving provides

118 Calories   51% Calories from Fat   7 g Fat
16 g Carbohydrates   1 g Protein   6 mg Calcium
0 g Dietary Fiber   16 mg Sodium   0 mg Cholesterol

Raspberry Sauce

7 servings
Serving size: 3 tablespoons.

Raspberry sauce has always been a classic accompaniment to many different desserts. Not only is it the ultimate flavor to pair up with deep dark chocolate, it seems to harmonize with such desserts as plain cheesecake or fresh berry tarts. Sometimes I prefer just to enjoy it over a scoop of vanilla ice cream or frozen yogurt. In this recipe I call for frozen berries because I can't bear to puree the fresh ones.

Ingredients

1 12-ounce package of frozen raspberries	1/4 cup granulated sugar
	1/4 cup water

Combine all ingredients in a medium-size saucepan and place over medium-high heat until berries are thawed and sugar is dissolved. Do not boil. Remove from heat and cool for 10 minutes. Strain mixture through a fine-mesh sieve to remove the seeds. Be sure to push as much of the berry pulp as possible through the sieve, otherwise the sauce will be too runny. A rubber spatula works well for this if you have a round sieve. If you are using a cone-shaped sieve, force the puree through with a small ladle.

Be sure to stir sauce before using it, since the pulp will separate from the liquid as the sauce settles. You can also make a thick raspberry sauce by adding 1 to 2 tablespoons of cornstarch to the strained sauce and cooking it in a saucepan over high heat until it reaches a boil and thickens, stirring occasionally. Start with a tablespoon of cornstarch, and if you want a thicker sauce, dissolve a little more in water and whisk it into the sauce while it is cooking. Cool sauce completely and store in an airtight container in the refrigerator. You can also freeze sauce. Serve cold.

Each serving provides

79 Calories   0% Calories from Fat   0 g Fat
21 g Carbohydrates   0 g Protein   8 mg Calcium
1 g Dietary Fiber   0 mg Sodium   0 mg Cholesterol

Strawberry Sauce

7 servings
Serving size: 3 tablespoons

Ingredients

1 pound fresh ripe straw-
  berries, stems removed
2 teaspoons fresh lemon
  juice

2 tablespoons granulated
  sugar

Combine all ingredients in a food processor fitted with the metal blade and puree until smooth. Strain mixture through a fine-mesh sieve to remove seeds. Be sure to push as much of the berry pulp as possible through the sieve. A rubber spatula works well for this if you have a round sieve. If you are using a cone-shaped sieve, force the puree through with a small ladle. Store in an airtight container in the refrigerator. You can also freeze the sauce. Be sure to stir the sauce before using, as the pulp separates from the liquid as the sauce settles. Serve cold.

Each serving provides

33 Calories   7% Calories from Fat   0.2 g Fat
8 g Carbohydrates   0 g Protein   9 mg Calcium
2 g Dietary Fiber   1 mg Sodium   0 mg Cholesterol

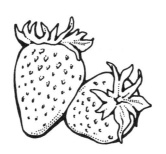

Orange Sauce

8 servings
Serving size: 3 tablespoons

This sauce is light and refreshing, and pairs up very nicely with fruit tarts and cheesecakes. It also adds a nice balance when served with chocolate desserts. If possible, squeeze fresh oranges for the best flavor; however, a good quality concentrate will also work well.

Ingredients

1½ cups orange juice, preferably fresh

1 tablespoon granulated sugar

2 teaspoons fresh lemon juice

2 tablespoons cornstarch

In a small saucepan combine all ingredients and whisk together until cornstarch has dissolved. Cook over high heat until sauce comes to a boil and thickens, stirring occasionally. Cool completely and store in an airtight container in the refrigerator. Serve cold.

Each serving provides

33 Calories   2% Calories from Fat   0.1 g Fat
8 g Carbohydrates   0 g Protein   4 mg Calcium
0 g Dietary Fiber   1 mg Sodium   0 mg Cholesterol

Sweet Deceptions

Apricot Puree

12 servings
Serving size: 2 tablespoons

This is not a thin, pourable sauce like the others—rather, it is thick and great to put in a squeeze bottle to pipe fancy designs all over the plate, or you can simply spoon some next to a dessert for a different flavor.

Ingredients

1 cup dried apricots
1 cup water

1/4 cup granulated sugar

Combine all ingredients in a small saucepan and cook over medium-high heat until apricots have absorbed most of the liquid. Cool completely and puree in a food processor fitted with the metal blade until smooth. When pureeing, you may have to add more water a tablespoon at a time to get the puree thick and smooth. If you would like a thinner sauce, you can thin it down with hot water. Store in an airtight container in the refrigerator. You can also freeze the puree. If you are using this puree to make the Lemon Apricot Pudding Cakes (page 140), do not thin it down any further; it should be the consistency of soft butter.

Each serving provides

47 Calories   1% Calories from Fat   0.1 g Fat
12 g Carbohydrates   1 g Protein   7 mg Calcium
1 g Dietary Fiber   2 mg Sodium   0 mg Cholesterol

Chocolate Ganache

Yield: about 1 cup
enough to frost two cakes

This dense, thick chocolate icing is used for frosting or filling some of the cakes in this book. You may want to frost other cakes or brownies as well. This recipe makes a generous amount of ganache; you can keep whatever you don't use in the refrigerator for up to a month.

Ingredients

1/4 cup liquid nondairy creamer

2/3 cup semisweet chocolate chips

In a small saucepan, heat the creamer over high heat until it reaches a boil. Remove from heat and add the chocolate chips. Let stand for a couple of minutes before stirring until smooth. If the chocolate has not melted completely, you can return it to the stove over medium heat and stir until it is melted and smooth. Cool completely before storing in an airtight container in the refrigerator.

To use, bring ganache to room temperature and use an icing spatula to spread on a cake or brownies. You may also heat it and pour it over a cake for a smooth chocolate coating.

Each serving provides

83 Calories   63% Calories from Fat   6 g Fat
9 g Carbohydrates   1 g Protein   5 mg Calcium
0 g Dietary Fiber   6 mg Sodium   0 mg Cholesterol

Sweet Deceptions

Chocolate Icing

Yield: ½ cup
enough to frost one cake

Not as heavy as the chocolate ganache, this icing is perfect to spread over a pan of brownies, or to drizzle over a cake.

Ingredients

1   cup powdered sugar
2   tablespoons unsweet-
    ened cocoa

2½   tablespoons milk
     (2 percent)

Combine all ingredients in a small bowl and stir until smooth and creamy. Spread icing over a pan of brownies, or drizzle it over a cake. You may add another teaspoon of milk for a thinner consistency.

Each serving provides

54 Calories   6% Calories from Fat   0 g Fat
13 g Carbohydrates   0 g Protein   8 mg Calcium
0 g Dietary Fiber   3 mg Sodium   0 mg Cholesterol

Crushed Meringue

A rustic yet very decadent touch when piled on top of cakes or even custards and tarts, this crisp meringue is light as a feather and adds a wonderful, crisp texture to desserts. The method requires nothing more than baking the meringue, then crumbling it into either large or small pieces. Then the ultimate finishing touch is to dust it with a coat of powdered sugar or cocoa, using a fine-mesh sieve.

Ingredients

3 large egg whites, at room temperature

1/8 teaspoon cream of tartar
1 cup granulated sugar

Line a cookie sheet with foil or parchment paper. Set oven on the lowest setting, which should be below 200 degrees F. In a medium-size mixing bowl that is clean and grease-free, beat the egg whites with the cream of tartar on medium speed of electric mixer until soft peaks form. Increase speed to high and sprinkle in the sugar, one tablespoon at a time, beating until all of the sugar has been incorporated and mixture is stiff and glossy. Use an icing spatula or rubber spatula to spread meringue onto prepared cookie sheet, 1/2-inch thick. It doesn't matter what it looks like because you're going to break it up. Place meringue in warm oven, and leave on overnight. This dries it out slowly, preserving its delicate, airy texture, and making the meringue crisp. When done, the meringue will be light beige and crisp all the way through. Cool the meringue for 10 minutes, then you may either break it up for decorating cakes and desserts, or store it in an airtight container at room temperature.

Variations

You can add many ingredients to the meringue before it goes into the oven to create different colors, flavors, and textures. These ingredients should be added once the meringue is stiff and glossy. Here are a few examples.

Chocolate meringue: Carefully fold 1/4 cup sifted unsweetened cocoa into the meringue, using a rubber spatula.

Nut meringue: Any kind of ground, toasted nut will do. Fold in 1/4 cup with a rubber spatula. Pistachios are especially pretty because of their color.

Chocolate chip meringue: Fold in 3/4 cup mini semisweet chocolate chips, or grated chocolate for a finer texture.

This recipe provides

97 Calories   0% Calories from Fat   0 g Fat
24 g Carbohydrates   1 g Protein   1 mg Calcium
0 g Dietary Fiber   35 mg Sodium   0 mg Cholesterol

Index

C

Cakes, *see also* Coffee cakes; Tarts;
    Tortes
  about, 21–22
  cardboard circles, 14
  cheese, *see* Cheesecakes
  cooling, 22–23
  devil's food with fudge icing, 54–55
  frozen toasted-almond mousse,
    138–139
  inverting, 22–23
  lemon apricot pudding, with blue-
    berry sauce, 140–141
  mixing batters, 22
  pans, *see specific types*
  peanut butter, tunnel of, 73–75
  pound, pear, 66–67
  short, strawberry amaretto, 68–69
  sponge, malted, 64–65
  storage, 28
  testers, 5
  transferring to platters, 23–24
  white chocolate raspberry revel,
    76–79
Cakey brownies, 98
  with creamy peanut butter icing, 99
Candy thermometer, 13
Caramel
  apple and walnut cobbler, 124–125
  coconut bars, 108–109
  crème, 132–133
  pecan and banana cheesecake,
    32–34
  pecan and coconut tart, 35–37
  sauce, gem, 200
  sauce, gooey, 198–199
Cardboard cake circles, 14
Carrot cake squares with cream cheese
    frosting, 106–107
Cheese, *see specific types*
  mascarpone, about, 15
  neufchâtel, about, 15
Cheesecakes
  caramel, pecan, and banana, 32–34
  chocolate malt, 38–39
  classic, 44–45
  lemon meringue, 59–61
  toasted hazelnut marble, 70–72
  unmolding, 25–27

Chef Mate, 9
Cherry
  almond bread pudding, 126–127
  cobbler muffins, 168–169
  pie filling, about, 16–17
Chocolate
  cinnamon muffins, 170
  crinkles, 88–89
  curls, preparing, 191–194
  death by, 49–53
  decor, 190–191
  ganache, 206
  icing, 207
  malt cheesecake, 38–39
  mousse, classic, 128–129
  peanut butter brownies, 100
  pistachio cookies, 94–95
  raspberry sanctuary, 40–41
  sauce, 201
  whiskey torte, 42–43
Chocolate Artistry, 192
Chocolate chip
  bread pudding, banana and, 121
  cookies, 86
  cookies, oatmeal and, 90–91
  muffins, 167
Cinnamon
  apple crunch muffins, 162–163
  chocolate, muffins, 170
  crunch muffins, 172–173
  swirl coffee cake, 180–181
Citrus cream cheese filling, berry tart
    with, 56–58
Classic cheesecake, 44–45
Classic chocolate mousse, 128–129
Cobblers
  blueberry peach, with cornmeal
    crisp, 150–151
  cherry, muffins, 168–169
  walnut, caramel apple and, 124–125
Cocoa, 194
Coconut
  bars, caramel, 108–109
  macaroon torte, 46–48
  pecan and coconut tart, 35–37
  raspberry macaroons, 87
Coffee, frozen, cream, 136–137
Coffee cakes, *see also* Cakes
  about, 160–161

frangipane coffee cake, 178–179
cinnamon swirl, 180–181
frosted spice, 184–185
Confectioners' sugar, *see* Powdered sugar
Cookies
apple raisin oatmeal bars, 104–105
baking temperature, 84–85
baking times, 84–85
cakey brownies, 98
with creamy peanut butter icing, 99
caramel coconut bars, 108–109
carrot cake squares with cream cheese frosting, 106–107
chocolate peanut butter, 100
chocolate chip, 86
dough, mixing, 2
fudgy brownies, 101
key lime squares, 110–111
luscious lemon squares, 112–113
measuring dough, 84
mixing dough, 84
oatmeal and chocolate chip, 90–91
PB & J kisses, 92–93
peanut butter, 114
pistachio chocolate, 94–95
sheets, 11–12
sugared hazelnut biscuits, 96–97
turtle brownies, 102–103
Cookie sheet, preparing, 83
Cooking spray, nonstick, 16
Cornmeal crisp, blueberry peach cobbler with, 150–151
Cottage cheese, about, 15
Cranberry bread, 182
Cream
frozen coffee, 136–137
Cream cheese frosting, carrot cake squares with, 106–107
Creamer, liquid nondairy, 15
Crème anglaise, 197
Crème brûlée with spiced rum, 130–131
Crème caramel, 132–133
Crushed meringue, 208–209
Cuisinart, 10
Custards
about, 117–118
baking, 118–119

banana flan, 122–123
crème brûlée with spiced rum, 130–131
crème caramel, 132–133
cups, 11
devil's food pots de crème, 134–135
vanilla, sauce, 197

D

Death by chocolate, 49–53
Desserts, cutting, hot-knife method, 5–6
Devil's food cake with fudge icing, 54–55
Devil's food pots de crème, 134–135

E

Egg
custard, about, 117–118
whites, preparing, 2–4
Electric mixer, 9–10

F

Fine-mesh sieve, 13
Flan, banana, 122–123
Flowers, edible, 195
Food processor, 10
Fresh berry tart with citrus cream cheese filling, 56–58
Frosted spice cake, 184–185
Frosting, *see also* Icing
cream cheese, carrot cake squares with, 106–107
Frozen coffee cream, 136–137
Fruits, fresh, 195
Fudge icing, devil's food cake with, 54–55
Fudgy brownies, 101

G

Gem caramel sauce, 200
Gingerbread loaves, 183
Ginger mousse, lemon, 142–143
Gonzalez, Elaine, 192
Gooey caramel sauce, 198–199

Nuts
  calorie content, 196
  toasted, 195–196

O

Oatmeal
  apple raisin bars, 104–105
  and chocolate chip cookies, 90–91
Orange
  almond, and poppyseed muffins, 174
  sauce, 204
Ovens, 4–5

P

Pans, *see specific types*
Parchment paper, 14
Paste, almond, 16
PB & J kisses, 92–93
Peach blueberry cobbler with cornmeal
    crisp, 150–151
Peanut butter
  about, 17
  cake, tunnel of, 73–75
  chocolate, brownies, 100
  cookies, 114
  creamy icing, cakey brownies
    with, 99
Pear pound cake, 66–67
Pecan
  caramel and banana cheesecake,
    32–34
  caramel and coconut tart, 35–37
Pies
  cherry filling, about, 16–17
  mud, *see* Mud pie, Sierra
Pistachio chocolate cookies, 94–95
Poppyseed
  almond and orange muffins, 174
  lemon, muffins, 171
Powdered malt, 17
Powdered sugar, 194
Praline, macadamia mousse, 144–146
Puddings, *see also* Bread
    puddings
  cake, lemon apricot, with blueberry
    sauce, 140–141
  molds, 11

Pumpkin spice muffins, 176–177
Pyrex-glass, 10

R

Raisin apple, oatmeal bars, 104–105
Raspberry
  chocolate sanctuary, 40–41
  coconut macaroons, 87
  lemon tart, 62–63
  mousse, 146
  sauce, 202
  white chocolate, revel, 76–79
Rice, arborio, 16
Rum, spiced, crème brûlè with, 130–131

S

Saran Wrap, 26–27
Saucepans, 12
Sauces
  apricot puree, 205
  blueberry, lemon apricot pudding
    cake with, 140–141
  chocolate, 201
  gem caramel, 200
  gooey caramel, 198–199
  orange, 204
  raspberry, 202
  strawberry, 203
  vanilla custard, 197
Shortcake, amaretto strawberry, 68–69
Sierra mud slide pie, 152–153
Sieves, *see* Fine-mesh sieve
Sour cream, 16
Spatulas, *see* Metal icing spatulas
Sponge cake, malted, 64–65
Springform pans, 11
Storage
  cakes, 28
  cookies, 85
  muffins, 160
Strawberry
  amaretto shortcakes, 68–69
  sauce, 203
Sugar, *see also* Powdered sugar
  adding to egg whites, 3
Sugared hazelnut biscuits, 96–97
Sultanas, 17

FILL IN AND MAIL TODAY

PRIMA PUBLISHING
P.O. Box 1260BK
Rocklin, CA 95677

USE YOUR VISA/MC AND ORDER BY PHONE
(916) 632-4400
Monday–Friday 9 A.M.–4 P.M. PST

I'd like to order copies of the following titles:

Quantity	Title	Amount
_____	*Sweet Deceptions* $14.95	_____
	Subtotal	_____
	Postage & Handling ($5 for first book, $0.50 for additional books)	_____
	7.25% Sales Tax (CA)	_____
	5% Sales Tax (IN and MD)	_____
	8.25% Sales Tax (TN)	_____
	TOTAL (U.S. funds only)	_____

Check enclosed for $_____ (payable to Prima Publishing)

HAWAII, CANADA, FOREIGN, AND PRIORITY REQUEST ORDERS, PLEASE CALL (916) 632-4400.

Charge my   ❑ MasterCard ❑ Visa

Account No. _____   Exp. Date _____

Print Your Name _____

Your Signature _____

Address _____

City/State/Zip _____

Daytime Telephone (___) _____